CW00631379

Botulinum To

Dirk Dressler

Foreword by Mitchell F. Brin

31 Figures
31 Tables

2000
Georg Thieme Verlag
Stuttgart · New York

Dr. Dirk Dressler
Department of Neurology
University of Rostock
Gehlsheimer Straße 20
18147 Rostock
Germany

*Die Deutsche Bibliothek –
CIP-Einheitsaufnahme*

Dressler, Dirk:
Botulinum toxin therapy : 31 tables /
Dirk Dressler. Foreword by Mitchell F. Brin.
– Stuttgart ; New York : Thieme, 2000
Dt. Ausg. u. d. T.: Dressler, Dirk:
Botulinum-Toxin-Therapie

© 2000 Georg Thieme Verlag
Rüdigerstraße 14
70469 Stuttgart, Germany

Printed in Germany

Cover design: Stefan Killinger,
  Kornwestheim
Graphics: Ziegler + Müller,
  Kirchentellinsfurt
Typesetting: Ziegler + Müller,
  Kirchentellinsfurt
  System: 3B2 (6.05)
Printing: Grammlich, Pliezhausen
Bookbinding: F. W. Held, Rottenburg

ISBN 3-13-117691-1 (GTV)
ISBN 0-86577-816-7 (TNY)

Important Note: Medicine is an ever-changing science undergoing continual development. Research and clinical experience are continually expanding our knowledge, in particular our knowledge of proper treatment and drug therapy. Insofar as this book mentions any dosage or application, readers may rest assured that the authors, editors, and publishers have made every effort to ensure that such references are in accordance with the **state of knowledge at the time of production of the book.**

Nevertheless, this does not involve, imply, or express any guarantee or responsibility on the part of the publishers in respect of any dosage instructions and forms of applications stated in the book. **Every user is requested** to examine carefully the manufacturers' leaflets accompanying each drug and to check, if necessary in consultation with a physician or specialist, whether the dosage schedules mentioned therein or the contraindications stated by the manufacturers differ from the statements made in the present book. Such examination is particularly important with drugs that are either rarely used or have been newly released on the market. **Every dosage schedule or every form of application used is entirely at the user's own risk and responsibility.** The authors and publishers request every user to report to the publishers any discrepancies or inaccuracies noticed.

Foreword

Alan Scott, M.D., was the first pioneer to explore the possibility that small doses of botulinum toxin type A (BT-A) could be safely injected directly into overactive muscles, reducing the intensity of muscle contraction. Since its introduction in the late 1970s for strabismus and the focal dystonia, blepharospasm, BT-A is being used successfully in the treatment of numerous other disorders characterized by excessive or inappropriate muscle contraction. These disorders include each form of focal dystonia; spasticity; inappropriate contraction in most of the body's sphincters, such as those associated with spasmodic dysphonia, achalasia, anal spasm, and vaginismus; eye movement disorders including nystagmus; other hyperkinetic disorders including tics and tremors; autonomic disorders such as hyperhidrosis; and cosmetically troublesome hyperfunctional facial lines (wrinkles). In addition, BT-A is being explored in the control of pain, with promising results in the management of myofascial pain syndrome, low back pain, tension and migraine headache.

As an example of physician and patient-driven research and discovery, this tremendous explosion in the use of a single agent to safely and effectively relieve chronic and heretofore often unmitigated human suffering is unparalleled in the history of medicine. It is a testimony to those physicians who, having recognized the potential of applying a controlled neuromuscular blockade, carefully tested this therapeutic in human subjects who equally accepted the opportunity, and often unknown risks, in an effort to advance medical knowledge and relieve symptoms of disease. For the most part, the discovery process was pioneered by people who seized the moment, and persevered.

Identification of new and novel uses of the toxin are limited by our own creativity and the ability to recognize a discovery, the therapeutic potential, and then systematically apply the principles of proof-of-concept, followed by controlled clinical trials. I am tantalized how each new therapeutic opportunity has brought new additional discoveries.

1. BT-A therapy has brought relief to patients with intractable muscle spasms and pain.
2. The realization of relief from suffering has returned patients into the therapeutic office, and into the major academic centers, also providing additional patients for clinical research. This, in the case of dystonia, has resulted in additional patients for genetic and pathophysiology studies. For instance, is dystonia really a motor disorder, or are the sensory feedback mechanisms potentially more important in the manifestations of disease?
3. Rare and orphan diseases are receiving additional attention. New funds from the government, private and industry sources have become available to explore the pathophysiology of diseases, and treatment options.
4. The observation that BT-A can treat primary pain disorders, such as migraine headache, is forcing a reassessment of the underlying pathophysiology of pain, in addition to a re-evaluation of the mechanism of action of neurotoxins.
5. Worldwide regulatory agencies have needed to develop specific protocols for the assessment, approval and monitoring of therapeutic toxin.

However, each new application brings additional challenges:
1. Physicians have to apply principles of *functional* anatomy so as to most effectively, skillfully and safely administer the toxin.
2. Medical, surgical and physical medicine specialties, along with allied health care workers such as speech and physical therapists, need to identify ways to work together in the common goal of providing symptomatic relief.
3. Patients need to be educated on the relative strengths, limitations and pitfalls of therapy so that expectations are appropriate and are realized during therapy.
4. Patient support organizations need to work interactively with health care providers in support of their constituencies.
5. Clinical scientists need to identify new methods to assess outcomes in the setting of clinical trials of novel therapeutics.

Dr. Dirk Dressler, an original BT pioneer, has written this guide to botulinum toxin therapy which is an incredible resource to health care providers, patients, and their families. Organized logically, composed interactively, and written in concise language with useful illustrations and tables, it provides a wealth of comprehensible information on the therapeutic application of BT-A and its mechanism of action. I am personally aware of the painstaking editing required for this single-authored volume, and it is a welcome addition to my clinic and practice.

Through the joint efforts of academic and industry scientists, the next phase of neurotoxin research and clinical applications is underway, with striking improvements in manufacturing techniques and the development of alternative serotypes for clinical use. Perhaps the most important advances will be the application of advanced toxin technology to the development of novel engineered toxins and therapeutics, which will be implemented as highly specific neuromodulators and therapeutic delivery vehicles.

New York
May 2000

Mitchell F. Brin, M.D.
Associate Professor of Neurology
Bachmann-Strauss Endowed Chair in Neurology
Mount Sinai School of Medicine
New York, NY, USA

Preface to the English Edition

I was rather pleased to see that this little book found quite a few readers since it was first published in German in 1995. I am even more delighted that Thieme Verlag is now prepared to produce an English version of it. Although it is based upon the original German version, it was updated, revised and substantially extended.

London   Dr. Dirk Dressler
July 1999

Preface to the German Edition

Botulinum toxin: the food poison, the biological weapon, the substance with the highest toxic potential of all natural and synthesised compounds...

These are not particularly promising features for a therapeutic use of a compound. On a closer look, however, this mysterious substance, of which nobody really knows why nature made it at all, reveals a completely different face: a delicate substance for highly specific blockade of cholinergic synapses, for producing a well controllable and focal muscle weakness and for blocking the vegetative innervation of glandular tissue.

So simple are these principles and so fascinating are botulinum toxin's potential applications in medicine– when only fantasy is allowed to stray.

The answers in this book are dedicated to all of those, who have not forgotten the simplest thing in life: to ask questions for curiosity's sake.

I would like to thank Dr. Klaus Geldsetzer for his valuable advise. I am also grateful to Dr. Petra Zwirner and the Deutsche Dystonie Gesellschaft e.V.

Schloss Berlepsch   Dr. Dirk Dressler
September 1995

Contents

Basic Principles of Botulinum Toxin Therapy

Properties of Botulinum Toxin

➤ What is BT known for traditionally?

Traditionally, BT is known as the substance with the highest specific potency of all natural or synthesised compounds. BT became infamous as the cause of botulism and as a biological weapon.

➤ What is botulism?

Botulism describes an intoxication with BT. Clinically, it is characterised by ocular impairment, such as double vision, blurred vision, ptosis, dilated and light-insensitive pupils, by gastrointestinal symptoms, such as dysphagia, nausea, vomiting, abdominal cramps and dry mouth, as well as, ultimately, paralysis of respiratory muscles and other localised or generalised pareses.

➤ How long has botulism been known to mankind?

Botulism has probably accompanied mankind since its beginning. In medieval times, it was known in Europe that production of sausages bears a high risk of food poisoning. Hence strict guild regulations had been imposed on sausage production and it may now be speculated whether, amongst other agents, also BT was involved in those food poisonings. In 1822 Justinus Kerner, a district physician in the state of Württemberg in the South West of Germany shown in Figure **1,** meticulously described the clinical picture of botulism, which was at that time endemic in this part of the country where large quantities of blood sausages were produced under inappropriate conditions on farms in the countryside. He, for the first time, linked the clinical pictures of botulism to BT. In 1895, Emile Pierre Marie van Ermengem investigated an outbreak of botulism in the small village of Ellezelles in Belgium and, for the first time, linked botulism with the germ *Clostridium botulinum.* In 1919, the existence of different BT types, then called A and B, became apparent. Later in the 1920's, Hermann Sommer of the Hooper Foundation at the University of California first concentrated BT-A into a relatively pure form. Today, botulism is monitored closely by governmental agencies all over the world. Improved hygienic standards have now virtually eradicated botulinism in industrialised nations. In the United States of America, only 215 outbreaks of food-borne botulism were recorded from 1950 to 1979.

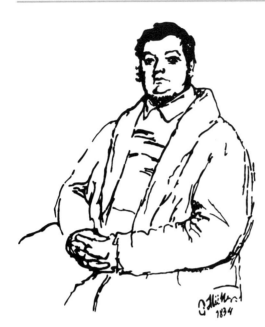

Fig. 1 Justinus Kerner (1786 – 1862). The German physician and poet published the earliest systematic description of food botulism. He was also the first to speculate on a possible therapeutic use of botulinum toxin.

Amongst animal populations, however, botulism epidemics still arise every once in a while, such as the one in the North Sea wetlands of Northwestern Germany, where some years ago large quantities of birds perished due to BT arising from decaying clams.

➤ **When was first speculated on the therapeutic use of BT ?**

It was Justinus Kerner who first speculated on the therapeutic use of BT in his famous monograph "Das Fettgift oder die Fettsäure und ihre Wirkungen auf den thierischen Organismus, ein Beytrag zur Untersuchung des in verdorbenen Würsten giftig wirkenden Stoffes" (The fat poison or the fatty acid and its effects on the animal organism, a contribution to the investigation of the substance which acts toxically in decayed sausages) published by Cotta in Stuttgart and Tübingen in 1822. In this book, he wondered whether BT, if applied in doses restricting its action to the sympathetic nervous system, could improve conditions he believed to originate from hyperexcitation of the sympathetic nervous system, such as St Vitus's dance now known as Huntington's chorea. Unfortunately, he did not pursue this line of thought and so his name is now still more famous for his poetry and for the grape named after him.

Later in the 1950's, Vernon B Brooks, a Canadian neurophysiologist, again raised the issue whether BT could be used to reduce muscle hyperactivity.

➤ What forms of botulism can be differentiated ?

The most common form of botulism is food botulism where the highly resistant spore form of *Clostridium botulinum,* which is distributed world-wide in soil and water, comes into contact with foods, such as sausages or vegetables. *Clostridium botulinum* is an obligate anaerobic, Gram-positive, rod-shaped organism. In older cultures it may also stain Gram-negative. The spore form of *Clostridium botulinum* is shown in Figure **2a.** Under exclusion of air and exposed to specific pH values, the spore form transforms into the vegetative form and produces BT, which may be ingested together with food and absorbed into the blood circulation. The vegetative form of *Clostridium botulinum* is shown in Figure **2b**. A less common form of botulism, first described in 1973, is wound botulism, where BT enters the blood circulation from wounds contaminated with *Clostridium botulinum.* In infant botulism, the gastrointestinal tract is colonised by *Clostridium botulinum,* which are constantly producing BT in situ. Infant botulism was first described in 1976.

➤ What is the role of BT as a biological weapon ?

Because of its extremely high toxic potential, BT has been investigated as a potential biological weapon by many military research laboratories since the second world war. This research provided much of the information which later facilitated the understanding of its therapeutic use. Although aerosols or BT poisoning of water supplies have been prepared – most recently during the Gulf war as shown in Figure **3** – BT has not been used in military conflicts so far. In some countries BT's association with biological warfare has considerably delayed its introduction as a therapeutic agent.

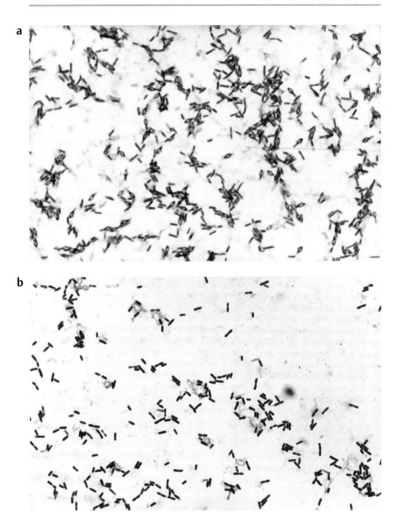

Fig. 2   *Clostridium botulinum* type F, Langeland strain. Brain-heart culture medium. **a** Spore form. 48 hours growth time. **b** Vegetative form. 12 hours growth time. Figures by courtesy of Ms H King and Dr HS Tranter, Public Health Laboratory Service, Centre for Applied Microbiology & Research, Salisbury, Wiltshire, UK.

A sick inventory

The agents of germ warfare fall into two categories: infectious diseases and biological toxins. The Iraqis developed both. Here is what they say they were working on:

Anthrax ....
....

Botulinum toxin. This is produced by the bacterium *Costridium botulinum.* It ist one of the most lethal substances known, killing by causing acute muscular paralysis. The incubation period and the prognosis both depend on the dose ingested. In severe cases, symptoms can set within four hours, and death follows swiftly. In all, Iraq claims to have produced 19,000 litres of concentrated botulinum toxin, of which al-

most 10,000 litres were put into munitions.

Aflatoxin ....
....

Gas gangrene ....
....

Wheat cover smut ....
....

Ricin ....
....

Viruses ....
....

Fig. 3 Recent report on the use of botulinum toxin as a biological weapon. From: The Economist 343 (8012/April 12th 1997): 111 – 114.

➤ **How did the therapeutic use of BT develop** ❓

For many years ophthalmologists had been seeking ways to avoid operations for strabismus by trying pharmacological blockades of external eye muscles. Various substances, such as alcohol, diisopropyl fluorophosphate and alpha-bungarotoxin, have been tested for this purpose. However, all of those substances failed because of intolerable side effects, such as painful inflammatory reactions, muscle necrosis, organotoxic side effects or insufficient duration of action. After years of animal experiments, BT was first used for strabismus by Dr AB Scott of the Smith Kettlewell Institute of Visual Sciences in San Francisco. Shortly afterwards, BT was used to treat blepharospasm. Since blepharospasm is in fact a focal dystonia, BT therapy was then rapidly adopted by neurologists and used in the treatment of various other forms of dystonia. Subsequently, it was employed in the treatment of other non-dystonic neurological conditions. Today, BT therapy finds its application in an ever increasing number of medical disciplines.

➤ **What is the structure of BT ?**

Both in its naturally occurring form and as a drug, BT consists of a mixture of various proteins. This mixture is shown in Figure **4**. The biologically active component of BT is BT neurotoxin which consists of two polypeptide chains with molecular masses of 50 kDalton and 100 kDalton. These two polypeptide chains are linked together by a single disulphide bond. Thus, BT neurotoxin is a complex and highly fragile macromolecule. Changes in pH value, exposure to light or heat induce conformational changes and finally destruction of the macromolecule with consecutive loss of its biological activity. BT neurotoxin is associated with various non-toxic proteins, some with haemagglutinating and some with non-haemagglutinating properties.

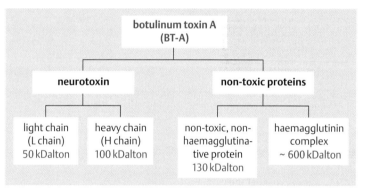

Fig. 4   Structure of botulinum toxin A (BT-A). BT-A consists of the neurotoxin, the biologically active component which is made up of a light chain and a heavy chain linked together by a single disulphide bond, and non-toxic proteins containing a haemagglutinin complex and non-haemagglutinative protein.

➤ **Are there different BT types ?**

To date, seven different types of BT are known and are designated by the letters A, B, C, D, E, F, and G.

➤ **What are the differences between the different BT types** ?

The different BT types differ slightly in the amino acid sequences of their neurotoxin and in their associated non-toxic proteins.

➤ **What is the exact structure of BT neurotoxin A** ?

The structure of BT-A has been studied extensively. Recently, the amino acid sequence of BT neurotoxin A was elucidated in detail. As shown in Figure **5,** it contains a total of 1296 amino acids, of which 848 form the heavy chain and 448 the light chain. Some uncertainties, however, still remain with regard to the spatial structure of BT neurotoxin.

```
M-P-F-V-N-K-Q-F-N-Y-K-D-P-V-N-G-V-D-I-A-Y-I-K-I-P-N-A-G-Q-M-Q-P-V-K-A-F-K-I-H-N-K-I-W-V-I-P-E-R-D-T-   (50)
F-T-N-P-E-E-G-D-L-N-P-P-P-E-A-K-Q-V-P-V-S-Y-Y-D-S-T-Y-L-S-T-D-N-E-K-D-N-Y-L-K-G-V-T-K-L-F-E-R-I-Y-S-  (100)
T-D-L-G-R-M-L-L-T-S-I-V-R-G-I-P-F-W-G-G-S-T-I-D-T-E-L-K-V-I-D-T-N-C-I-N-V-I-Q-P-D-G-S-Y-R-S-E-E-L-N-  (150)
L-V-I-I-G-P-S-A-D-I-I-Q-F-E-C-K-S-F-G-H-E-V-L-N-L-T-R-N-G-Y-G-S-T-Q-Y-I-R-F-S-P-D-F-T-F-G-F-E-E-S-L-  (200)
E-V-D-T-N-P-L-L-G-A-G-K-F-A-T-D-P-A-V-T-L-A-H-E-L-I-H-A-G-H-R-L-Y-G-I-A-I-N-P-N-R-V-F-K-V-N-T-N-A-Y-  (250)
Y-E-M-S-G-L-E-V-S-F-E-E-L-R-T-F-G-G-H-D-A-K-F-I-D-S-L-Q-E-N-E-F-R-L-Y-Y-Y-N-K-F-K-D-I-A-S-T-L-N-K-A-  (300)
K-S-I-V-G-T-T-A-S-L-Q-Y-M-K-N-V-F-K-E-K-Y-L-L-S-E-D-T-S-G-K-F-S-V-D-K-L-K-F-D-K-L-Y-K-M-L-T-E-I-Y-T-  (350)
E-D-N-F-V-K-F-F-K-V-L-N-R-K-T-Y-L-N-F-D-K-A-V-F-K-I-N-I-V-P-K-V-N-Y-T-I-Y-D-G-F-N-L-R-N-T-N-L-A-A-N-  (400)
F-N-G-Q-N-T-E-I-N-N-M-N-F-T-K-L-K-N-F-T-G-L-F-E-F-Y-K-L-L-C-V-R-G-I-I-T-S-K-T-K-S-L-D-K-G-Y-N-K-↓-A-L-  (450)
N-D-L-C-I-K-V-N-N-W-D-L-F-F-S-P-S-E-D-N-F-T-N-D-L-N-K-G-E-E-I-T-S-D-T-N-I-E-A-A-E-E-N-I-S-L-D-L-I-Q-  (500)
Q-Y-Y-L-T-F-N-F-D-N-E-P-E-N-I-S-I-E-N-L-S-S-D-I-I-G-Q-L-E-L-M-P-N-I-E-R-F-P-N-G-K-K-Y-E-L-D-K-Y-T-M-  (550)
F-H-Y-L-R-A-Q-E-F-E-H-G-K-S-R-I-A-L-T-N-S-V-N-E-A-L-L-N-P-S-R-V-Y-T-F-F-S-S-D-Y-V-K-K-V-N-K-A-T-E-A-  (600)
A-M-F-L-G-W-V-E-Q-L-V-Y-D-F-T-D-E-T-S-E-V-S-T-T-D-K-I-A-D-I-T-I-I-I-P-Y-I-G-P-A-L-N-I-G-N-M-L-Y-K-D-  (650)
D-F-V-G-A-L-I-F-S-G-A-V-I-L-L-E-F-I-P-E-I-A-I-P-V-L-G-T-F-A-L-V-S-Y-I-A-N-K-V-L-T-V-Q-T-I-D-N-A-L-S-  (700)
K-R-N-E-K-W-D-E-V-Y-K-Y-I-V-T-N-W-L-A-K-V-N-T-Q-I-D-L-I-R-K-K-M-K-E-A-L-E-N-Q-A-E-A-T-K-A-I-I-N-Y-Q-  (750)
Y-N-Q-Y-T-E-E-E-K-N-N-I-N-F-N-I-D-D-L-S-S-K-L-N-E-S-I-N-K-A-M-I-N-I-N-K-F-L-N-Q-C-S-V-S-Y-L-M-N-S-M-  (800)
I-P-Y-G-V-K-R-L-E-D-F-D-A-S-L-K-D-A-L-L-K-Y-I-Y-D-N-R-G-T-L-I-G-Q-V-D-R-L-K-D-K-V-N-N-T-L-S-T-D-I-P-  (850)
F-Q-L-S-K-Y-V-D-N-Q-R-L-L-S-T-F-T-E-Y-I-K-N-I-I-N-T-S-I-L-N-L-R-Y-E-S-N-H-L-I-D-L-S-R-Y-A-S-K-I-N-I-  (900)
G-S-K-V-N-F-D-P-I-D-K-N-Q-I-Q-L-F-N-L-E-S-S-K-I-E-V-I-L-K-N-A-I-V-Y-N-S-M-Y-E-N-F-S-T-S-F-W-I-R-I-P-  (950)
K-Y-F-N-S-I-S-L-N-N-E-Y-T-I-I-N-C-M-E-N-N-S-G-W-K-V-S-L-N-Y-G-E-I-I-W-T-L-Q-D-T-Q-E-I-K-Q-R-V-V-F-K- (1000)
Y-S-Q-M-I-N-I-S-D-Y-I-N-R-W-I-F-V-T-I-T-N-N-R-L-N-N-S-K-I-Y-I-N-G-R-L-I-D-Q-K-P-I-S-N-L-G-N-I-H-A-S- (1050)
N-N-I-M-F-K-L-D-G-C-R-D-T-H-R-Y-I-W-I-K-Y-F-N-L-F-D-K-E-L-N-E-K-E-I-K-D-L-Y-D-N-Q-S-N-S-G-I-L-K-D-F- (1100)
W-G-D-Y-L-Q-Y-D-K-P-Y-Y-M-L-N-L-Y-D-P-N-K-Y-V-D-V-N-N-V-G-I-R-G-Y-M-Y-L-K-G-P-R-G-S-V-M-T-T-N-I-Y-L- (1150)
N-S-S-L-Y-R-G-T-K-F-I-I-K-K-Y-A-S-G-N-K-D-N-I-V-R-N-N-D-R-V-Y-I-N-V-V-V-K-N-K-E-Y-R-L-A-T-N-A-S-Q-A- (1200)
G-V-E-K-I-L-S-A-L-E-I-P-D-V-G-N-L-S-Q-V-V-V-M-K-S-K-N-D-Q-G-I-T-N-K-C-K-M-N-L-Q-D-N-N-G-N-D-I-G-F-I- (1250)
G-F-H-Q-F-N-N-I-A-K-L-V-A-S-N-W-Y-N-R-Q-I-E-R-S-S-R-T-L-G-C-S-W-E-F-I-P-V-D-D-G-W-G-E-R-P-L* (1296)
```

Fig. 5 Amino acid sequence of botulinum neurotoxin A. The entire amino acid sequence consists of 1296 amino acids, of which 848 amino acids constitute the heavy chain of the neurotoxin. The light chain consists of 448 amino acids. From: Binz T, Kurazono H, Wille M, Frevert J, Wernars K, Niemann H (1990) The complete sequence of botulinum neurotoxin A and comparison with other clostridial neurotoxins. J Biol Chem 265: 9153 – 9158.

➤ **Do all BT types use the same mechanism of action** ?

All seven BT types bind to the same glycoprotein structures and hence they all block the cholinergic synapse. The BT types differ, however, in their intracellular mechanism of action, since they link to different components of the acetylcholine vesicle transport system.

➤ **Why is BT-A the most suitable BT type for therapeutic use ?**

Probably caused by different intracellular mechanisms of action, BT-A has a particularly long duration of action. It is also easy to produce and has a favourable ratio between biologically active and inactive BT neurotoxin.

➤ **Are other BT types being tested for possible therapeutic use ?**

Other BT types are being tested for therapeutic use. Trials with BT-F and BT-B are the most advanced. BT-F and BT-B have already been used experimentally on a number of patients. While BT-B will probably be introduced as a drug under the name NeuroBloc® in the near future, this is questionable for BT-F.

➤ **Are special preparations of BT-A being tested for possible use ?**

It is believed that BT-A preparations in which the non-toxic protein fraction has been removed will soon be tested for therapeutic use. These highly purified BT-A preparations may have substantial advantages over conventional preparations because of their lower antigenicity.

Mechanism of Action of Botulinum Toxin

➤ **What is the clinical action of BT ?**

Clinically, BT induces a blockade of the cholinergic innervation of the target tissue. Thus, the target tissue is chemically denervated by BT. When BT is administered into muscle tissue, paresis results. The degree of this paresis can be well controlled by the amount of BT administered. Additionally, the so induced paresis is almost exclusively limited to the target muscle. Thus, after administration into muscle tissue, BT acts as a well controllable local muscle relaxant. When BT is administered into glandular tissue, blockade of the parasympathetic and – in some tissues the sympathetic – innervation results. Again, this blockade can be controlled effectively and is limited predominantly to the target tissue. Thus, after administration into glandular tissue, BT serves as a well controllable local parasympatholytic or sympatholytic agent.

➤ What is the site of action of BT ?

When BT is injected into a target tissue, it is almost completely bound to acceptor structures. These acceptors consist of glycoproteins and are found exclusively on cholinergic nerve endings. Thus, BT expresses its activity exclusively at cholinergic nerve endings.

➤ In what target tissues has BT been used therapeutically so far ?

So far, BT has been used almost exclusively in muscle tissue, where it acts on the cholinergic neuromuscular synapse. However, BT has just recently also been used in glandular tissue, where it acts on the cholinergic parasympathetic or cholinergic sympathetic synapse.

➤ How does BT act on cholinergic synapses ?

The mode of action of BT is illustrated in Figure **6**. BT neurotoxin binds with its heavy chain to BT acceptors on cholinergic nerve endings. Sub-

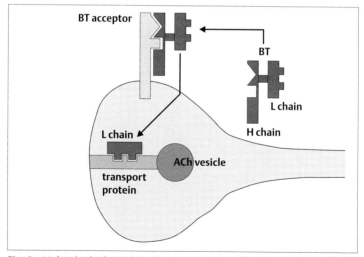

Fig. 6 Molecular-biological mechanism of action of botulinum toxin (BT). BT neurotoxin binds with its H chain to the BT receptor on the cholinergic nerve ending. Subsequently, the L chain of BT neurotoxin is transported into the cholinergic nerve ending where it blocks the transport molecules mediating the transport of acetylcholine vesicles to the synapse.

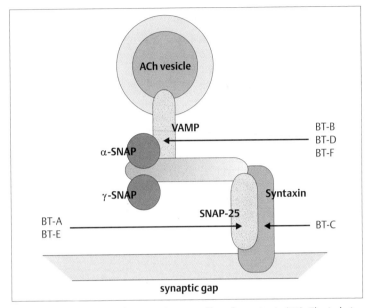

Fig. 7 Intracellular mechanism of action of botulinum toxin (BT). The L chains of the different BT neurotoxin types proteolytically cleave the various proteins mediating the transport of acetylcholine vesicles to the synapses. Modified from: Barinaga M (1993) Secrets of secretion revealed. Science 260: 487–489.

BT-A	L chain of BT neurotoxin A
BT-B	L chain of BT neurotoxin B
BT-C	L chain of BT neurotoxin C
BT-D	L chain of BT neurotoxin D
BT-E	L chain of BT neurotoxin E
BT-F	L chain of BT neurotoxin F
NSF	N-ethylmaleimide-sensitive factor
α-SNAP	soluble NSF attachment protein type α
γ-SNAP	soluble NSF attachment protein type γ
SNAP-25	synaptosomal-associated protein of 25 kDa
VAMP	vesicle-associated membrane protein (= synaptobrevin)

sequently, the light chain is transported into the nerve ending. Inside the nerve ending, the light chain protolytically blocks proteins transporting the acetylcholine vesicles to the cell wall. This blockade of the transport molecules is shown in Figure **7**.

➤ **How long does the blockade of the
acetylcholine transport protein last ?**

The blockade of the acetylcholine transport proteins is believed to be irreversible. This is an essential prerequisite for the therapeutic use of BT, since it assures a sufficient duration of action of the BT therapy.

➤ **How is the action of BT within the target tissue terminated ?**

The action of BT within the target tissue is terminated by axonal sprouting of the peripheral nerve. These axons form new fully functional synapses re-innervating the target tissue. Recently, it was argued whether the action of BT within the target tissue is determined by prolonged intracellular presence of the intact BT within the peripheral nerve terminal. Then axonal sprouting would merely be an epiphenomenon.

➤ **How long does it usually take before re-innervation
of the target tissue can be detected clinically ?**

It normally requires about three months before clinical re-innervation of the target tissue occurs. Re-innervation of the target tissue is complete after about another two months. So far, no substantial differences in the re-innervation time of different target muscles have been observed. This suggests that the re-innervation process is localised in the distal parts of the peripheral nerve only.

➤ **How often does re-innervation occur after
BT-induced denervation of the target tissue ?**

After repeated use of BT in muscle tissue, which for some indications can now be followed over a period of more than 10 years, between 30 and 50 re-innervations have been observed without occurrence of any persisting denervations.

➤ **What is the therapeutic window ?**

The term therapeutic window describes the suitability of a target muscle for BT therapy for dystonia. In a target muscle, dystonic strength and voluntary strength can be distinguished. Voluntary strength, in turn, consists of functional strength and reserve strength. Functional strength describes the minimal strength needed to maintain physiological functioning under conditions of normal use. Reserve strength is the strength that is needed only under conditions of exceptional use. The objective of BT therapy is to reduce dystonic strength as much as possible. However, by doing this voluntary strength is reduced to the same extent. Thus, if BT therapy is to be used without occurrence of functional impairment under normal use, the reduction of voluntary strength must remain within the range of reserve strength. Thus, reserve strength determines the width of the therapeutic window for the target muscle. These relationships are shown in Figure **8.**

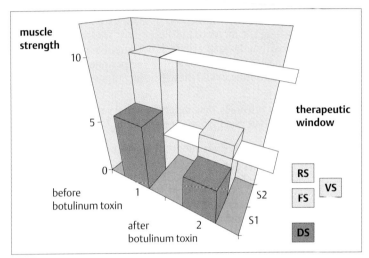

Fig. 8 Therapeutic window. The term therapeutic window describes the suitability of a target muscle for botulinum toxin (BT) therapy of dystonia. In the target muscle dystonic strength (DS) and voluntary strength (VS) can be distinguished. VS consists of functional strength (FS) and reserve strength (RS). FS describes the strength necessary to maintain physiological functioning of the target muscle under conditions of normal use. RS is the strength that is required only under conditions of exceptional use. The objective of BT therapy is to reduce DS as much as possible. However, VS is concomitantly reduced to the same extent as DS. Thus, if BT therapy is to be used without functional deficits under normal use, reduction of VS must remain within the range of the RS.

➤ **Is the width of the therapeutic window
the same in different target muscles ?**

The width of the therapeutic window is different in different target muscles. This is shown in Table **1**. Interestingly, clinical observations of patients with botulism show that certain muscles respond to systemic application of BT with higher sensitivity than others, suggesting different reserve strengths as the underlying cause.

Table 1   Width of the therapeutic window in various target muscles

width of therapeutic window	muscle
wide	orbicularis oculi
medium	neck muscles axial muscles
narrow	finger extensors finger flexors muscles of the corner of the mouth

➤ **What other factors determine the suitability
of a target muscle for BT therapy ?**

In addition to the width of the therapeutic window, the anatomic position of the target muscle influences its accessibility and thus its suitability for BT therapy. For example, access to prevertebral neck muscles is severely restricted limiting their suitability for BT therapy. The anatomic proximity of the target muscle to muscles which could elicit problematic side effects in case of BT diffusion also limits its suitability. This is, for example, the case with hyoid muscles situated adjacent to pharyngeal and oesophageal muscles, which can produce swallowing difficulties when infiltrated by aberrant BT.

➤ **What are the advantages of BT over other substances
used for chemical denervation of muscle tissue ?**

Under normal circumstances, therapeutic BT doses do not produce intolerable or even dangerous side effects. Local tissue irritation or muscle necrosis is not observed. BT does not produce organotoxic side effects and it remains almost completely within the target muscle. The therapeutic effect can be well controlled and lasts for a sufficient period of time.

Side Effects of Botulinum Toxin

➤ **How can the side effects of BT therapy be classified ?**

The side effects of BT therapy can be divided into obligatory side effects and facultative side effects. The facultative side effects can be further subdivided into local and systemic ones.

➤ **What are the obligatory side effects of BT therapy ?**

Depending on the extent to which the innervation of the target tissue has to be blocked to achieve the therapeutic effect, physiological functioning of the target tissue is always reduced accordingly. In muscle tissue this produces paresis of the target muscle. However, in most cases this paresis will not impair normal functioning, because many muscles possess a sufficiently wide therapeutic window and agonistic muscles can, at least partly, take over the function of the target muscle. So far, obligatory side effects have not been observed in glandular tissue, since in these conditions a primary hyperactivation is reduced to a physiological level.

➤ **What are the facultative side effects of BT therapy ?**

Local side effects can occur during BT therapy when BT diffuses from the target tissue into adjacent tissues. Here BT can cause temporary impairment of muscle and glandular tissues. However, this impairment is relatively short-lasting, since it is caused by fractions of the BT administered. The frequency of local side effects depends on the amount of BT injected and also on the consistency of the target tissue. Systemic side effects can occur when BT is washed out of the target tissue or when it is accidentally injected into blood vessels.

➤ **Have any side effects been caused by the non-toxic proteins ?**

No side effects have been caused by the non-toxic proteins so far. In very rare cases, administration of BT has been accompanied by short flu-like symptoms. However, it remains unclear whether these symptoms are related to BT therapy at all and, if so, whether they represent systemic side effects of BT or immunological reactions. The haemagglutinative properties of the non-toxic proteins occur in vitro only.

Safety Aspects of Botulinum Toxin Therapy

➤ Why is BT therapy not hazardous for patients ?

BT therapy is not hazardous for patients because the total dose of BT administered for therapeutic purposes is only a fraction of the BT dose required to cause dangerous systemic side effects. Additionally, therapeutic doses of BT are given strictly intramuscularly where they remain bound to acceptor structures. BT not bound to these acceptors is probably degraded within a few hours.

➤ What is the long-term experience with the use of BT therapy ?

BT therapy has been used since about 1980 in many thousands of patients. A number of these patients have received more than 50 injection series. In 1993 alone, about 130 000 vials of BT were used for therapeutic purposes world-wide and today this number should have increased substantially.

➤ Does BT therapy cause organ damage ?

No evidence for organ damage caused by BT therapy has been reported so far. Organ damage resulting from BT therapy is unlikely to occur since BT remains almost entirely within the target tissue and is not distributed systemically.

➤ What changes occur in the target muscle after repeated administration of BT ?

After repeated BT administration dystonic muscle hypertrophy of the target muscle can be reduced. Necrotic changes or fibrotic changes of the target muscle have not been observed.

➤ Is BT distributed systemically after intramuscular administration ?

When low or moderate BT doses are administered, about 5% of the intramuscularly injected BT will be distributed systemically. On administration of higher BT doses, this proportion may increase rapidly due to the limited binding capacity of the BT acceptors. This may be important when high BT doses are given in a small number of target muscles. High BT dosages should therefore be given with caution. If used at all, they should be built up gradually over several injection series.

➤ How can systemically distributed BT be detected ?

Systemically distributed BT cannot be detected directly because the amounts involved are below the detection threshold of physical analytical methods. Single fibre electromyography, a very sensitive method for investigating neuromuscular transmission, however, can detect discrete changes in neuromuscular transmission of muscles distant from the BT injection sites.

➤ Are there any systemic side effects of BT therapy ?

Because of the high intramuscular binding of BT, systemic side effects of BT therapy are very rare. If they do occur, they only occur after administration of very high BT doses, which may occasionally be necessary in exceptional cases. Generalised weakness, fatigue, shortness of breath, dysphagia, perspiration fits and accommodation difficulties may then occur. In most cases, these side effects last for a few days only. Accidental intravascular injections have not been reported so far.

➤ Why does BT normally not induce an immune response ?

For therapeutic purposes, only minute amounts of BT are administered. It is believed that these amounts are too low to stimulate the immune system. Additionally, BT is administered strictly intramuscularly so that immunologically competent body tissues are not exposed to BT.

➤ Can BT induce impairment of the central nervous system ?

BT cannot induce direct impairment of the central nervous system because, as a macromolecule with a molecular weight of 150 kDalton, it cannot penetrate the blood brain barrier.

➤ Is BT transported within the peripheral nerve into the spinal cord ?

Autoradiographic studies show that BT is transported into the spinal cord along the peripheral nerve innervating the target muscle. This process is known as retrograde axonal transport.

➤ **Does the retrograde axonal BT transport
  cause damage to the peripheral nerve?**

Neurographic investigations have shown that the retrograde axonal BT transport does not damage the function of the peripheral nerve. It is assumed that BT is degraded during its retrograde axonal transport.

➤ **Is BT transported transsynaptically within
  the central nervous system?**

Retrograde axonal transport ends in the soma of the motor neuron. Transsynaptic transport to spinal interneurons, Renshaw cells or other central nervous system structures has not been demonstrated.

➤ **Does BT cause allergic complications?**

Allergic complications, such as urticaria, oedema or cardiovascular reactions, have not been observed. Allergic reactions are unlikely because of the low BT doses used for therapy. Recently, a small sample of patients was reported who received BT for cervical dystonia and subsequently developed a clinical picture resembling transient neuralgic shoulder amyotrophy. In retrospect, this was similar to an early report of a patient who developed polyradiculoneuritis in a somewhat loose temporal relationship to BT treatment. However, the nature of these phenomena and their causal relationship to BT administrations remain unclear.

➤ **Are there interactions between BT and other drugs?**

Concomitant administration of calcium antagonists may inactivate BT. In patients with long-standing administration of corticosteroids and consecutive myopathy, increased BT sensitivity should be suspected. Simultaneous administration of glycoside antibiotics may result in potentiation of the effects of BT.

➤ **What patients should be excluded from BT therapy?**

BT therapy should not be used in patients with impairment of neuromuscular transmission such as Lambert-Eaton syndrome or myasthenia gravis. Pregnant women should also not undergo BT therapy for the time being. Patients with impaired haemostasis should be treated with special attention to avoid haemorrhage.

➤ **Is BT harmful to the embryo or foetus?**

So far, there have been only few documented cases of accidental use of BT during pregnancy. In these cases embryonic and foetal development were without complications. Since BT is a macromolecule that cannot pass through the placenta, embryonic or foetal damage seems unlikely. Teratogenicity studies performed with rats and mice tend to support this assumption.

➤ **What are the highest single BT doses employed so far in BT therapy?**

In some of our patients with severe generalised dystonia, the highest single doses of BT employed were about 800 mouse units Botox®. In these cases BT doses were built up gradually within two or three injection series. The use of such high doses should be reserved for exceptional circumstances. By no means is it advisable to administer such large amounts as an initial single dose.

Failure of Botulinum Toxin Therapy

➤ **How can BT therapy failure be described?**

BT therapy failure can be described according to clinical features and according to results of technical investigations.

➤ **What are the clinical features of BT therapy failure?**

Clinically, BT therapy failure can be described as primary or secondary. Primary therapy failure means failure of BT therapy on its first use in a patient. Unfortunately, there is no general consensus as to how many attempts have to be made before primary therapy failure has to be concluded. Secondary therapy failure means failure of BT therapy after its initially successful use. Therapy failure may also be described as partial or complete, objective or subjective, and temporary or permanent.

➤ **How can BT therapy failure be documented?**

BT therapy failure can be documented by neurological examination testing target muscle paresis and target muscle atrophy, by clinical rating scales, standardised video protocols and by treatment calendars. A treatment calendar based upon the patient's self assessment is shown in Figure **9** (Appendix, p. 128). Despite its subjectivity, this treatment calendar reflects the patient's condition over the full treatment period rather than just the short and usually artificial situation when the patient is seen by the physician. Special clinical rating scales and video protocols will be presented in the sections describing particular conditions treated with BT therapy.

➤ What technical investigations can be used to evaluate BT therapy failure?

BT therapy failure can be evaluated by EMG testing and by BT antibody testing.

➤ How is EMG testing for evaluation of BT therapy failure performed?

EMG testing for evaluation of BT therapy failure investigates the BT induced reduction of EMG activity in a target muscle in a suspect patient and compares this reduction to the reduction measured in a control population. EMG testing therefore investigates the basic mechanism of BT's therapeutic action directly within a target muscle.

For EMG testing the maximal voluntary activation of the sternocleidomastoid muscle is measured before BT administration and two weeks after BT administration by using surface recording electrodes. If the BT induced reduction of the maximal voluntary activation is less than the reduction seen in a control population when the same amount of BT is administered, the result of the EMG test is pathological. Figures **10** and **11** show reference dose-effect graphs for the application of Botox® and Dysport® in the sternocleidomastoid muscle.

EMG testing can be performed on the sternocleidomastoid muscle easily since it is readily identified, since it allows reproducible electrode positions and since it is frequently involved in cervical dystonia so that additional BT administrations can be avoided. Physiological activation of the target muscle avoids electric stimulation which is often unpleasant for the patient.

➤ How can BT antibodies be detected?

BT antibodies can be detected by the mouse protection bioassay in which the test serum together with a specific amount of BT is administered to a group of mice. If there are more survivors in this group of

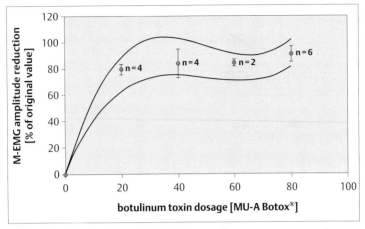

Fig. 10   Reference dose-effect graph for Botox® administration into the sternocleidomastoid muscle. Botox® (100 MU-A in 2.5 ml 0.9% NaCl/H$_2$0) is administered into 3 injection sites equally distributed over the muscle belly. Surface EMG measurements under maximal voluntary activation were performed before and 2 weeks after botulinum toxin administration. Curves are polynomial trend curves (n = 3, Microsoft Excel version 5.0) of the doubled standard deviations.

n   number of injected muscles
MU-A   mouse units of the mouse bioassay of Allergan Inc
⊕   mean value plus and minus doubled standard deviation

mice than to be expected from the BT dose given without the test serum, the test serum contains neutralising antibodies as a protective factor.

. Recently, the mouse diaphragm bioassay has been introduced in which a mouse hemidiaphragm is fixed to a force measurement device and repetitively stimulated through the phrenic nerve, the time between BT administration and occurrence of half-maximal diaphragm paralysis is then measured. If the test serum contains BT antibodies, this paralysis time is prolonged in relation to the amount of BT antibodies contained in the test serum.

Trials with ELISA tests to detect BT antibody formation have also been performed for some time. For this test highly purified BT is fixated on a static medium. BT antibodies contained in the test serum are bound to the static medium and can be visualised by a detection reagent.

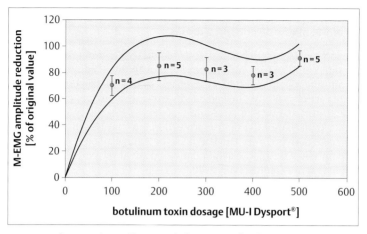

Fig. 11 Reference dose-effect graph for Dysport® administration into the sternocleidomastoid muscle. Dysport® (500 MU-I in 2.5 ml 0.9 % NaCl/H₂0) is administered into 3 injection sites equally distributed over the muscle belly. Surface EMG measurements under maximal voluntary activation were performed before and 2 weeks after botulinum toxin administration. Curves are polynomial trend curves (n = 3, Microsoft Excel version 5.0) of the doubled standard deviations.

n	number of injected muscles
MU-I	mouse unit of the mouse bioassay of Ipsen Ltd
⊖	mean value plus and minus doubled standard deviation

➤ **What are the advantages and disadvantages of the mouse lethality bioassay ?**

The mouse protection bioassay tests the neutralising activity of BT antibodies, thus monitoring a property closely related to BT therapy. Disadvantages are the large number of animals sacrificed, the personnel costs, and the time delay before the result of the test can be obtained. The mice sacrificed in this test are exposed to prolonged suffering over several days. Furthermore, quantification of the results is difficult. At present, the mouse protection bioassay is not commercially available.

➤ **What are the advantages and disadvantages
  of the mouse diaphragm bioassay ?**

The mouse diaphragm bioassay tests blockade of neuromuscular transmission by BT and its impairment by neutralising BT antibodies, thus monitoring a parameter directly related to BT's therapeutic effect. Its results are quantitative, involve sacrifice of one mouse per two tests only, and can be available after a few hours. Its sensitivity seems to be higher than that of the mouse protection bioassay. Disadvantages are the costs deriving from the specialised equipment necessary and the preparation of the mouse diaphragms. At present the mouse diaphragm bioassay is not commercially available either.

➤ **What are the advantages and disadvantages of the ELISA test ?**

The ELISA test for detection of BT antibodies is cheaper than the mouse bioassays, can be performed quickly, and does not involve sacrifice of animals. Thus it is highly suitable for epidemiological studies on the development of BT antibodies. The results of the ELISA test are quantitative. A disadvantage is that BT antibodies binding to BT but not influencing its bioactivity cannot be distinguished from neutralising BT antibodies. The test sensitivity necessary for the detection of the extremely low BT antibody titres has not yet been achieved. The BT antibody test is also not yet commercially available.

➤ **What is the role of BT antibody testing
  in the evaluation of BT therapy failure ?**

The use of BT antibody testing for evaluation of BT therapy failure is limited since results obtained with BT antibody testing are contradictory. Using the mouse protection bioassay, BT antibodies are detected in most cases of secondary therapy failure, whereas, in some others, they are not detected. Conversely, in most patients without BT therapy failure, BT antibodies are not detected, whereas, in some others, they are detected. The mouse diaphragm bioassay seems to be more sensitive than the mouse protection bioassay. As yet, experience with ELISA tests in patients with BT antibodies is limited.

➤ How often does BT therapy failure occur in the treatment of dystonia ?

Reports on BT therapy failure in cases of dystonia are rare. Since definitions of primary and secondary therapy failure have not yet been generally accepted and since most cases of therapy failure have neither been objectified nor quantified, these reports must be interpreted with caution. The frequency of therapy failures depends on the condition treated. For treatment of cranial and cervical dystonia, the frequencies of primary and secondary therapy failures should be in the region of about 1 to 5 % each. Information on the frequency of therapy failures using BT therapy for other indications is still lacking.

➤ What are the causes of primary BT therapy failure ?

There are many causes of primary therapy failure. As with all other therapies, the clinical condition for which the therapy is intended to be used has to be diagnosed properly. For most conditions where BT therapy is indicated there are differential diagnoses which do not respond to BT therapy. Clinical subtypes with a limited response to BT therapy exist for most conditions. Full biological activity of the BT drug applied is necessary as well. Exact planning of BT therapy, consisting of identification of appropriate target muscles and appropriate BT doses, is essential and has to be performed for each patient individually. Primary therapy failure can be due to difficulties in the exact administration of BT into the target muscle. Other possible causes, such as the existence of pre-formed, cross-reacting tetanus toxin antibodies, presence of acceptor variants or cellular immune responses are hypothetical so far.

➤ How can primary BT therapy failure be evaluated ?

Figure **12** shows a flow diagram for evaluation of primary therapy failure. After establishing a diminished response to BT therapy clinically, the most important step in this process is EMG testing. An exact neurological examination can determine whether untreatable differential diagnoses or clinical subtypes with reduced sensitivity to BT therapy are present. Controls of the BT administration technique, the biological activity of the BT drug, BT antibody testing and careful evaluation of the patient's history help to identify causes of primary therapy failure.

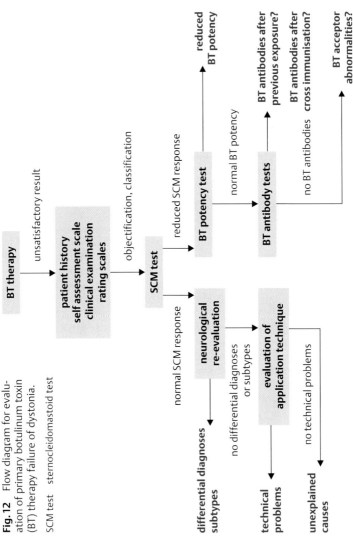

Fig. 12 Flow diagram for evaluation of primary botulinum toxin (BT) therapy failure of dystonia.

SCM test   sternocleidomastoid test

➤ **What are the causes of secondary therapy failure?**

Like primary therapy failure, secondary therapy failure may also be caused by various factors. It may be due to a worsening of the original symptomatology even though such exacerbations after a prolonged, stable course of the disease are not frequent in dystonia. Psychological factors may influence the patient's perception of the treatment outcome. It is frequently seen that the first BT administration is considered by the patient to be especially effective. Technical problems with the injection of BT into the target muscle may also give rise to secondary therapy failure. If a reduced response of the target muscles to BT is noted, this may be due to a reduced biological activity of the BT drug or the formation of BT antibodies. Changes in BT acceptors or cellular immune responses are hypothetical so far.

➤ **How can secondary BT therapy failure be evaluated?**

Figure **13** shows a flow diagram for evaluation of secondary therapy failure. Again, after secondary decrease of the response to BT therapy is established clinically, EMG testing is the most important step. Video controls, psychological examinations and checks of the BT administration technique and the biological BT activity as well as BT antibody testing should be carried out additionally.

➤ **How often does BT antibody formation occur during BT therapy?**

In general, the frequency of BT antibody formation during BT therapy is probably overestimated. During BT therapy for cranial dystonia, not a single case of BT antibody formation has been reported in the literature so far, despite the long-standing experience with this indication. According to present knowledge, approximately 5% of patients treated for cervical dystonia respond with BT antibody formation. For indications where high BT doses are required, however, the proportion of patients with BT antibody formation appears to be higher. Studies about the prevalence of BT antibody formation including all relevant aetiologic factors are still lacking.

➤ **How can BT antibody formation be suspected clinically?**

First of all, a clear reduction of the outcome of BT therapy has to be established, either by the patient or the physician or by both. For this purpose clinical scales may be used, although they are usually not sensitive

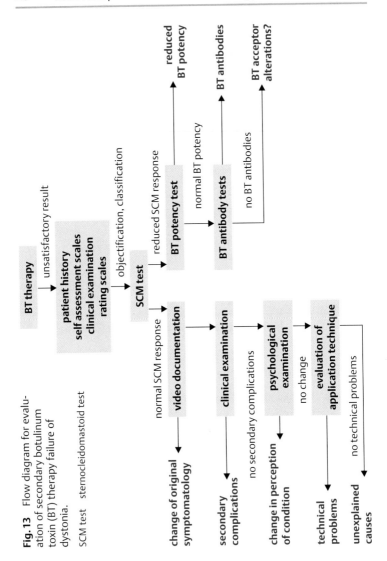

Fig. 13 Flow diagram for evaluation of secondary botulinum toxin (BT) therapy failure of dystonia.

SCM test   sternocleidomastoid test

enough. A self-assessment scale is more sensitive but includes subjective factors. Usually, BT antibody formation occurs within 200 to 1100 days after initiation of BT therapy. However, late therapy failures can occur. Figure **14** shows the spectrum of latencies between initiation of BT therapy and occurrence of complete secondary BT therapy failure. BT antibody formation is usually preceded by injection series with partially reduced therapeutic effect. This partial reduction can consist of reduced maximal therapeutic effect, reduced duration of the therapeutic effect, or both. A prolonged latency until the onset of the therapeutic effect is rare, but may occur as well. Table **2** shows the clinical features of secondary BT therapy failure suggestive of BT antibody formation.

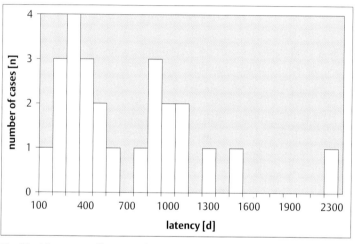

Fig. 14 Histogram of latencies between initiation of botulinum toxin therapy and occurrence of complete secondary therapy failure.

➤ **What are the factors influencing formation of BT antibodies?**

When groups of patients with suspected BT antibody formation are compared with groups of patients with normal responses to BT the risk factors shown in Table **3** can be identified. BT antibody formation depends on the size of the BT doses used. Although formation of BT antibodies took place in one patient treated by us for cranial dystonia, there are no reports in the literature on BT antibody formation for this indication so far. Antibody formation has only been reported in cases where

Table 2   Clinical features of secondary botulinum toxin therapy failure suggestive of antibody formation

complete loss of improvement on two or more consecutive botulinum toxin applications
("complete secondary therapy failure")

partial loss of improvement prior to complete secondary therapy failure
("preceding partial secondary therapy failure")

EMG reduction in SCM test more than 2 standard deviations below EMG reduction in control population
("pathological SCM test")

exclusion of other causes of subjective or objective botulinum toxin therapy failure

Table 3   Risk factors for formation of botulinum toxin antibodies

high single doses of botulinum toxin

short intervals between injection series

repeated botulinum toxin injections within less than 2 weeks
("booster injections")

female sex?

BT dosages were several-fold higher than the dosages usually used for cranial dystonia. BT antibody formation is inversely related to the length of the interval between injection series. BT injections given at intervals of less than two weeks ("booster injections") increase the risk of BT antibody formation. It remains unclear so far how strong the individual or combined influence of these risk factors on the occurrence of BT antibody formation is. From analogies with immunisation experiments against BT, the individual response of the patient's immune system may be considerably more important than all other risk factors.

➤ How long should the interval between injection series be ?

The interval between injection series should be at least two months to avoid excessive stimulation of the immune system with consecutive risk of BT antibody formation. Since detailed epidemiological data on BT antibody formation are lacking, this recommendation is currently entirely arbitrary. However, most of the physicians using BT would agree with this interval. It is still a matter of some controversy whether additional BT administration ("booster injections") is justified in order to optimise the therapy effect at the beginning of the treatment. With sufficient experience this additional BT administration should not be necessary. However, if booster injections are performed, an interval of seven to ten days after the initial BT administration is optimal. Undesired cumulative effects can occur when shorter intervals are used while longer intervals lead to a unfavourable fragmentation of the BT effect.

➤ **What is the role of the non-toxic BT proteins in BT therapy failure ?**

The non-toxic BT proteins do not seem to play a role in BT therapy failure. They dissociate from BT neurotoxin on reconstitution of the BT drug. If antibodies would be formed against non-toxic BT proteins, they would not antagonise the therapeutic effect of BT.

➤ **What is the further management of patients with complete secondary BT therapy failure with pathological EMG test ?**

Until the results of BT antibody testing can be interpreted appropriately, complete secondary BT therapy failure with pathological EMG testing should be considered as being due to BT antibody formation, even if BT antibody testing – especially with the mouse protection bioassay – is negative. Further BT administration should be stopped for the time being. Only sparse information is available on the persistence of BT antibody titres over time. From analogies with immunisation experiments against BT, there is a chance that, if further BT exposure is avoided, BT antibody titres will decrease spontaneously. However, whether BT toxoid used for the immunisation experiments and unattenuated BT as used for BT therapy have the same antigenic properties remains unclear. In our experience there are indications that BT antibody titres slowly decrease, but within one year after cessation of BT administration normal EMG responses were not regained. Even if time intervals of one year would be acceptable for patients, it remains unclear whether renewed BT exposure would not cause an immediate increase of the BT antibody titres. At the moment it seems that under these circumstances the spectrum of conventional treatment options will have to be employed.

➤ Can BT therapy failure caused by BT antibody formation be overcome by using increased BT doses?

Initially, BT therapy failure caused by BT antibodies may be overcome by increased BT doses as long as the BT antibody titres are low. However, increased BT doses are likely to induce formation of even more BT antibodies and finally this ends in a dead race between increased BT doses and increased BT antibody titres. Whether there are patients existing with partial secondary BT therapy failure and only slightly increased BT antibody titres that can be treated on a long term basis with moderately increased BT doses, remains unclear for the time being.

➤ Can additional administration of immunosuppressants antagonise the action of BT antibodies?

Additional administration of immunosuppressants around the time of BT administration did not prevent the BT inactivation by BT antibodies in a sample of our patients. More aggressive regimens of immunomodulation have not been tried so far.

➤ Can BT antibodies be extracted from the blood of patients with BT therapy failure?

In principle, BT antibodies might be extracted from the blood of patients with BT therapy failure by means of plasmapheresis, immunoabsorption, and intravenous administration of immunoglobulin. However, none of these techniques has been tried so far in these patients.

➤ Can the administration of other BT types be helpful in cases of BT therapy failures caused by BT-A antibodies?

There does not seem to be any cross-reactivity of BT antibodies against different BT types. Antibodies which are able to inactivate BT-A, thus do not seem to cause inactivation of other BT types. Administration of different BT types in cases of BT-A antibody-induced therapy failure could, in principle, be helpful. In fact, first experience with the administration of BT-F and BT-B in patients with BT-A antibodies has produced a normal therapeutic response. However, long-term experience with this strategy is not available. If formation of BT antibodies does indeed depend mainly on the reactivity of the patient's immune system, subsequent production of antibodies against BT-F or BT-B can be expected.

At present, BT-F and BT-B are neither authorised for use in humans nor are they generally available.

Botulinum Toxin Drugs

➤ **How are BT drugs produced** ?

BT drugs are produced biologically. *Clostridium botulinum* from a controlled breeding strain with a high yield of BT production is incubated in a fermenter under exclusion of air and using specific nutrition media, temperatures and pH conditions. After about 36 hours the *Clostridium botulinum* culture has achieved maximum growth and cytolytic processes activated by extracellular proteases start to liberate intracellular BT precursors into the culture medium. After about 72 hours, the maximum BT concentration is reached and the culture is killed off by addition of acid. After centrifugation, the BT is subjected to various purification processes, that had long been known, but had to be modified for the production of BT drugs to prevent toxic contaminations. These purification processes consist of a series of precipitation reactions and ion-exchange chromatographies. At the end of these processes, when about half of the original BT content has been lost, sterile, highly purified BT neurotoxin bound to non-toxic proteins is isolated. The purity of the product can be confirmed by photometric and electrophoretic methods. Finally, the product is subjected to the most important step, the pharmaceutical formulation. Here, the biological activity of each BT batch is determined by mouse lethality bioassay and standard solutions are prepared by adding saline (Botox®) or lactose solution (Dysport®) which is also necessary for protection of BT's steric conformation during lyophilisation. For prevention of surface absorption human serum albumin is added. To achieve long term stability during storage the water content is extracted by lyophilisation (Dysport®) or by another method (Botox®).

➤ **What are the main components of BT drugs** ?

BT drugs consist of BT neurotoxin A, non-toxic proteins, human serum albumin and traces of lactose or saline solution.

➤ **What BT drugs are currently commercially available** ?

BT drugs currently commercially available are produced by two pharmaceutical companies. Allergan Inc of Irvine, California, USA is marketing a BT drug under the trade name Botox® and Ipsen Ltd of Maidenhead, Berkshire, UK, is distributing a BT drug under the trade name Dysport®. Both BT drugs are shown in Figure **15**. Elan Pharmaceuticals of San Francisco, California, USA is currently performing clinical trials to register a BT-B product under the trade name NeuroBloc™. Whether companies in countries such as China are planning to produce BT for therapeutic use, is not known.

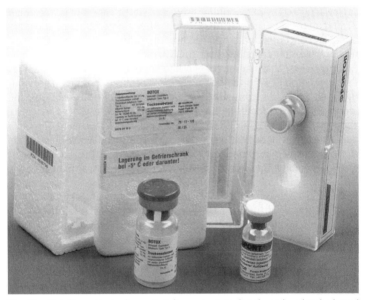

Fig. 15   Botulinum toxin drugs. Botulinum toxin is distributed under the brand names Botox® (Allergan Inc) and Dysport® (Ipsen Ltd).

➤ **Are there any differences between the two commercially available BT drugs ?**

Since both BT drugs are based on BT-A there are no principle differences in their modes of action. Because of the different manufacturing processes, there are slight differences in the non-toxic protein content, the auxiliary substances and the specific biological activity. However, no differences in their therapeutic actions have been noticed so far.

➤ **How is the biological activity of BT determined ?**

The biological activity of BT is measured in mouse units. One mouse unit corresponds to the LD_{50} value for BT in a specific mouse population. For determination of this LD_{50} value different BT doses are administered to groups of Swiss Webster mice. A dose-response curve is constructed from the mortality rates of the individual groups and, from this curve, the BT dose can be calculated at which 50 % of a given mouse population would have died.

➤ **Is it useful to measure therapeutic BT dosages in weight units ?**

It is not useful to measure therapeutic BT dosages in weight units. The appropriate parameter is the biological activity measured by the mouse lethality bioassay and given in mouse units. The biological activity can change because of steric changes resulting, for example, from ageing processes, which would not be detected in the weight of the sample. Weight measurements can often be misleading when it is not clear to which portion of the BT preparation they are referring.

➤ **What is the biological activity of the two commercially available BT drugs ?**

The biological activities of the two BT drugs as given by the manufacturers are 100 mouse units for one vial of Botox® and 500 mouse units for one vial of Dysport®.

➤ **Can the biological activity of both BT drugs be compared on the basis of the biological activity given by the manufacturers ?**

The biological activity of both BT drugs cannot be compared on the basis of the data given by the manufacturers. The reason for this are probably differences in the mouse lethality bioassays used by the manufacturers. Reliable measurements of both BT drugs with one mouse lethality assay are surprisingly not available.

Handling of Botulinum Toxin Drugs

➤ **In which two forms do BT drugs exist ?**

BT drugs exist in an unreconstituted and in a reconstituted form. The unreconstituted form refers to the freeze-dried BT drug, while the reconstituted form refers to the BT drug dissolved and diluted in physiological saline.

➤ **How should unreconstituted BT drugs be transported and stored ?**

Unreconstituted BT drugs should be transported and stored only under cooling. For Botox® the recommended storage temperature is – 5 °C and for Dysport® it is between + 4 and + 8 °C. Recent experiments have shown that short-term exposure to higher storage temperatures should not lead to a significant loss of biological activity. It is likely that the registration and licensing authorities will soon allow higher storage temperatures. At temperatures of more than 30 °C rapid inactivation takes place.

➤ **How long can unreconstituted BT drugs be stored under approved conditions ?**

The storage times approved by registration and licensing authorities as from completion of production are 24 months for Botox® and 9 months for Dysport®. The expiry date of the respective batch is printed on each vial. Recent experiments have shown that a marked decrease in the strength of action is not to be expected after longer storage under approved conditions. Again, it is to be expected that the approved storage times will be extended by registration and licensing authorities in the near future.

➤ **How are BT drugs reconstituted?**

The BT drugs are reconstituted by addition of sterile and non-preserved physiological saline (0.9 % NaCl/H_2O). The concentration of the BT drug is determined by the amount of saline added.

➤ **What mistakes can be made when reconstituting BT drugs?**

In most countries, saline preparations with different concentrations are delivered in containers with similar appearances. Quite frequently, these different containers are stored in the same place as well. Therefore, there is always a risk that BT drugs are reconstituted with saline of the wrong concentration. If this happens, BT injections are accompanied by prolonged pain, either when too low or when too high concentrations are used. At this point the suspicion may arise whether anecdotal reports of painful BT injections may not be caused by use of inappropriate saline concentrations.

➤ **Are the therapeutic effects of BT influenced by the concentration of the BT drugs?**

It can be assumed that reconstitution of a given amount of BT with higher volumes of saline increases penetration of BT within the target tissue and vice versa. It can also be assumed that increased BT penetration changes the therapeutic outcome by either producing a more widespread paresis or by producing more collateral spread into adjacent muscles thus inducing higher rates of side effects.

➤ **What concentration of BT drugs should be used?**

Experiments investigating optimal dilutions of BT drugs have not yet been performed. One way of addressing this problem is to decide on an practical injection volume and then add the necessary amount of BT. Reasonable injection volumes for mid-sized muscles, such as neck muscles, are in the order of 0.5 to 2.0 ml. Assuming then dosages for these muscles in the order of 20 to 80 mouse units Botox® gives a dilution of 100 mouse units Botox® in 2.5 ml 0.9 % NaCl/H_2O. From our experience this dilution seems to be suitable for most purposes. Higher concentrations can be necessary for the administration of higher BT doses in facial regions in order to avoid too large injection volumes. We have found it quite helpful to use a standard dilution wherever possible to improve intuitive dosing by remembering volumes rather than abstract mouse units.

➤ How should the reconstituted BT drugs be handled ?

Reconstituted BT drugs are more sensitive to environmental influences than the unreconstituted product. They should not be exposed to direct sunlight or higher temperatures. Careful shaking of the vials to reconstitute the BT drugs is preferable over reconstitution using syringes where high pressures can build up on forcing the liquid through under-dimensioned cannulas and thus risking mechanical denaturation.

➤ Can reconstituted BT drugs be refrozen ?

Reconstituted BT drugs cannot be refrozen without risking denaturation, since the sensitive molecular structure of BT can be damaged by crystallisation on slow, undried freezing.

➤ How long can reconstituted BT drugs be stored ?

Due to the fragility of the disulphide bond between the heavy chain and the light chain of the BT neurotoxin, reconstituted BT drugs can only be stored for a few hours. They should be used within 2 to 3 hours.

➤ Why is the handling of BT drugs unproblematic ?

Unreconstituted BT drugs are biologically inactive. Reconstituted BT drugs have a relatively short life-time. This short life-time can be seen as an "inherited self-destruction tendency". Therefore, laboratory contaminations with BT are not critical. Additionally, BT contaminations can quickly and easily be inactivated by chemical disinfection. Thus, elaborate safety measures are not required for handling of BT drugs.

➤ How can BT drugs be disposed of safely ?

Disposal of reconstituted BT drugs is not a safety problem since, due to their inherited self destruction tendency, their biological activity is lost within a few hours. Special treatment of BT vials as hazardous waste is not necessary.

Clinical Applications of Botulinum Toxin Therapy

Dystonia

➤ What is dystonia ?

The term dystonia describes a specific form of involuntary muscle hyperactivity. Dystonic muscle hyperactivity is defined as "sustained and frequently causing twisting and repetitive movements or abnormal postures" (Ad Hoc Committee of the Dystonia Medical Research Foundation, 1984).

➤ Is dystonia a disease or a syndrome ?

The term dystonia describes a syndrome. Dystonia may be caused by many different diseases and conditions.

➤ How can dystonia be classified ?

Dystonia can be classified according to the categories listed in Table **4.** The most frequently used category is the distribution of dystonia within the body. This classification is helpful as an indicator of severity and can also be a help for planning therapeutic strategies. Classification according to the aetiology is also frequently used. This classification is especially useful for the understanding of dystonia, for therapeutic considerations, and for genetic counselling.

Other classifications referring to the patient's age at onset, morphology of the dystonic muscle hyperactivity, the conditions of their occurrence, the continuity of their occurrence, and the localisation of the first symptoms are usually used only for special purposes.

➤ What is primary dystonia ?

The term primary dystonia describes conditions where dystonia is the sole symptom. Under this definition occurrence of tremor is allowed, as long as it is not clear whether this dystonic tremor represents an independent entity. Primary dystonia covers the vast majority of all dystonias.

Table 4   Classification of dystonia according to different categories

category	feature	subgroup	cause
distribution	cranial	blepharospasm	
		oromandibular	
	cervical	torticollis	
		laterocollis	
		ante-/retrocollis	
	pharyngolaryngeal		
	axial		
	limbs		
	segmental		
	generalised		
	hemidystonia		
aetiology	primary	familial	Oppenheim's dystonia (DYT1-gene at 9q34), others
			sporadic
	secondary	drugs	neuroleptics (acute or chronic), levodopa (chronic), others
		trauma	central nervous system, peripheral nervous system
		hypoxia	
		haemorrhage, infarction	
		infection (acute, post-infectious conditions)	
		tumours	
		intoxications	
		dystonia plus	dopa responsive dystonia (gene defect for GTP cyclohydroxylase I at 14q22.1)
			myoclonic dystonia

Table 4 Classification of dystonia according to different categories   *(continuation)*

category	feature	subgroup	cause
		heredodegenerative	Lubag (DYT3-gene defect at Xq13)
			Huntington's disease (IT15-gene defect at 4 p 16.3)
			Wilson's disease (gene defect for Cu-ATPase at 13 q14.3)
			Leigh's disease (gene defect in mitochondrial DNA)
			cortico-basal ganglionic degeneration
			progressive supranuclear palsy
			Parkinson's disease
age of onset	adulthood		
	childhood		
morphology	tonic		
	clonic		
	tremulous		
	fixed		
conditions of occurrence	spontaneous		
	action-induced		
	stress-induced		
continuity of occurrence	continuous		
	intermittent		
	paroxysmal		
localisation of first symptoms	legs		
	non-legs		

➤ What is secondary dystonia?

The term secondary dystonia describes conditions where dystonia can be attributed to endogenous or exogenous noxa. These noxa are numerous. In principle, all noxa that can damage appropriate structures of the nervous system can cause dystonia.

➤ What are dystonia plus syndromes?

The term dystonia plus syndrome describes conditions where dystonia is associated with other, non-heredodegenerative symptoms. Dystonia plus syndromes are very rare.

➤ What is heredodegenerative dystonia?

The term heredodegenerative dystonia describes conditions where dystonia is associated – and probably caused – by heredodegenerative disorders. Heredodegenerative dystonia is also a rare condition, since only a small minority of dystonias is associated with heredodegenerative conditions and only few heredodegenerative conditions elicit dystonic features.

➤ Is dystonia an organic or psychogenic condition?

Today it is generally accepted that dystonia is an organic condition. However, like other organic conditions, it can be modulated by numerous psychological factors. It is still not clear whether unusual psychological stress can contribute to the manifestation of an otherwise subclinical dystonia.

➤ In which part of the central nervous system are lesions localised that can cause dystonia?

In patients with dystonia lesions of the basal ganglia can occasionally be identified. These lesions are localised most frequently in the putamen. It is assumed that damage in various parts of the complexly interlinked basal ganglia can lead to dystonia. Sometimes lesions can be found within the brain stem. Lesions within the spinal cord or even within the peripheral nervous system have been controversially discussed. However, with the currently available diagnostic tools, pathological findings cannot be detected in about 90% of the patients suffering from dystonia.

➤ Is there a pathophysiological model for dystonia ?

Attempts have been made to develop a pathophysiological model of dystonia by using the basal ganglia scheme of Alexander and Crutcher. Using data from animal experiments and from positron emission tomography, it seems that in dystonia there is a neuronal hyperactivity of the direct and possibly the indirect pathways connecting the putamen and the internal part of the globus pallidus. This is shown in Figure **16.**

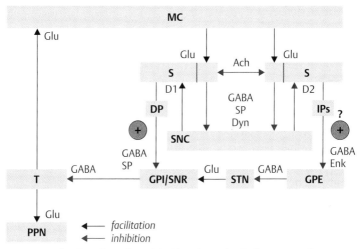

Fig. 16 Pathophysiological model of basal ganglia dysfunction in dystonia. It is hypothesised that dystonia originates from neuronal hyperactivity in the direct striatopallidal pathway and possibly in the indirect striatopallidal pathways. Modified from: Hallett M (1993) Physiology of basal ganglia disorders: an overview. Can J Neurol Sci 20: 177 – 183 and Alexander GE, Crutcher MD (1990) Functional architecture of basal ganglia circuits: neural substrates of parallel processing. Trends Neurosci 13: 266 – 271.

Ach	acetylcholine	MC	motor cortex
D1	dopamine receptor type 1	PPN	pedunculopontine nucleus
D2	dopamine receptor type 2	S	striatum
DP	direct pathway	SNC	substantia nigra,
Dyn	dynorphin		pars compacta
Enk	enkephalin	SNR	substantia nigra,
GABA	gamma-aminobutyric acid		pars reticulata
Glu	glutamate	SP	substance P
GPE	globus pallidum, external part	STN	subthalamic nucleus
GPI	globus pallidum, internal part	T	thalamus
IPs	indirect pathways		

➤ **In which parts of the body is dystonia most frequently localised ?**

Dystonia is most frequently localised in the eyelid closing muscles. Dystonia of the neck muscles is probably equally common. Limb dystonia is less common, although the frequency of limb dystonia after cerebral infarction is not well documented. Rare forms of dystonia are laryngeal dystonia and generalised dystonia.

➤ **What is the prevalence of dystonia**
   within the general population ?

Unfortunately there are no reliable data available on the prevalence of dystonia within the general population. The available figures originate from the time prior to the introduction of BT therapy and are tainted by various methodological problems. It is assumed that there are about 80 patients with dystonia per 100 000 members of the general population. Thus, there should be about 70 000 dystonia patients in Germany and more than 200 000 dystonia patients in the United States of America. The corresponding figures for Parkinson's disease are between 85 and 187 per 100 000 members of the general population and for multiple sclerosis in Central Europe about 200 per 100 000 members of the general population. Despite vigorous efforts by patient organisations to increase awareness of dystonia and despite growing interest in dystonia within the neurological profession dystonia is still underdiagnosed to a substantial extent.

➤ **What are the conventional treatment options for dystonia ?**

The conventional treatment options for dystonia are summarised in Table **5.** Drug therapy on the whole has been disappointing. At most, one third of the patients improve, when the whole set of drug regimens are tried. Additionally, these improvements are almost always partial and restricted to a limited period of time. Side effects are frequent and often lead to discontinuation of the therapy. The general opinion is that trihexyphenidyl (Artane®) is the substance of first choice. Second choice drugs include tetrabenazine, clonazepam, baclofen, tizanidine, haloperidol, or lisuride. The number of other drugs with therapeutic effects on a single case basis is legion.

   Surgical treatments are also limited by partial success and – depending on the technique applied – possible side effects. In denervation procedures, re-innervation processes and repair processes in connective tissues can result in re-occurrence of the initial symptomatology after a relatively short period of time. However, denervation procedures probably offer the second best choice for patients in whom BT therapy has failed and drug therapy is unsatisfactory.

Physiotherapy can help to prevent secondary complications of dystonia. In BT therapy for cervical dystonia it can help to re-adjust the head position reflexes and to strengthen muscles acting as antagonists to dystonic muscles. Relaxation techniques can offer a short lasting relief and are best used in situations of acute dystonia exacerbation.

➤ **Does BT have a specific effect against dystonia ?**

According to current knowledge, BT exerts its therapeutic effect on dystonia solely by blocking cholinergic neuromuscular synapses. Since these synapses transmit not only dystonic nerve impulses but also nerve impulses of voluntary movements, BT does not reduce dystonic muscle activity selectively. Furthermore, there is no autoradiographic evidence for BT reaching postsynaptic spinal or supraspinal structures which could be involved in mediation or generation of dystonia. Recent findings indicating a BT effect on muscle spindles seem to reflect epiphenomena.

➤ **How can dystonia be documented ?**

Dystonia can be evaluated by video recording. Table **6** (Appendix, p. 130) shows a standardised video protocol for this purpose. Dystonic movements and dystonia induced disability can be documented with the rating scales shown in Tables **7** (Appendix, p. 132) and **8** (Appendix, p. 134). Treatment calendars as shown in Figure **9** (Appendix, p. 128) allow a long-term follow-up of the condition. Based upon the patient's self-assessment they are, however, subjective.

➤ **What are the difficulties in evaluating the therapy effects on dystonia ?**

Dystonia induces distortion and malpositioning of body parts with functional impairment and frequently pain sensation. Distortion and malpositioning of body parts can – at least in principle – be objectified by angle measurements. However, intermittent measurements are hardly adequate to describe dystonic symptoms which can vary widely with time. This is also the case with measurements of functional impairment. Data on pain sensation must be purely subjective. Their correlation with visible portions of the dystonic symptomatology is limited.

Table 5 Conventional treatment options for dystonia

treatment acting peripherally

physiotherapy	fango
	massages
	balneotherapy
	short wave therapy
peripheral surgery	muscle transsection
	peripheral nerve transsection
	posterior ramisectomy
	rhizotomy (anterior or posterior)
	nerve decompression

treatment acting centrally

relaxation techniques	autogenic training, biofeedback
spinal antispastic agents	baclofen (oral, intrathecal)
	tizanidine
	lisuride
	clonazepam
central surgery	stereotactic procedures
	spinal cord stimulation
central nervous system agents	anticholinergic agents
	benzhexol/trihexyphenidyl
	biperidene

Table 5 Conventional treatment options for dystonia *(continuation)*

treatment acting centrally	*(continuation)*		
	dopamine antagonists	classic neuroleptics	perphenazin pimozide haloperidol
		tetrabenazine reserpine benzamides	tiapride sulpiride
	dopamine agonists	L-DOPA bromocriptine MAO-B inhibitors	
	membrane stabilisers	carbamazepine lithium	
	beta blockers	propranolol	

➤ **Is a purely somatic therapy sufficient
for the treatment of dystonia ?**

As with most chronic disorders, purely somatic therapy is not sufficient
in most patients suffering from dystonia. Somatic therapy should be accompanied by psychotherapeutic and social support. Many patients
have expressed the opinion that this aspect of dystonia treatment is often neglected.

➤ **What psychological problems may be caused by dystonia ?**

At the onset of the condition, the patient frequently suffers from a loss
of self-confidence. Typically the patient's mood alternates between the
hope for remission and the realisation that chances for this are limited.
Later, fears about a progression of the condition may be experienced.
These fears concern both the severity of the symptomatology as well
as the spread of the symptomatology. The longer the diagnosis is delayed, the more the patient's confidence in the medical profession is
put at risk. In this situation, some patients with severe dystonia can develop suicidal ideas. Social impairment becomes more obvious the
more the condition progresses. Typically, the patient withdraws from
his or her environment, sometimes to the extent of complete isolation.
This social withdrawal is the result of the often stigmatising nature of
the condition, the first functional impairment, and the lack of understanding in the environment. Inferiority complexes and depressive reactions are not infrequent and, in turn, increase the tendency for withdrawal even further. Finally, a vicious circle develops which may be
hard to break. Depending on the degree to which the patient's environment becomes accustomed to the dystonic symptomatology, the situation usually de-escalates to some extent. However, in more severe cases
normal social contacts are only seldom regained. In advanced stages of
the condition loss of employment and long-term hospitalisations can
change the life style dramatically. Resignation often arises at this stage.

➤ **What forms of psychological help can be
offered to patients with dystonia ?**

A marked improvement in the psychological condition of the patient
can usually be achieved by offering information about the disorder to
those in closer contact with the patient. Helping the patient with pre-
formulating a short but clear explanation of the disorder for those in
the patient's wider social environment is also usually helpful. The pa-

tient's living conditions should be analysed and strategies developed in order to avoid specific psychological and physical stress situations. Discussions together with members of the patient's family can offer the patient positive perspectives for planning the future with the disorder.

➤ What social problems can be caused by dystonia ?

The most difficult social problem is the lack of understanding in the social environment about the nature and the cause of the disorder. This is not surprising considering the lack of information the patients and the sometimes even their physicians suffer from. Because of the unique nature of the symptoms, psychological disorders are often assumed to be the cause of dystonia. Quite frequently suspicions about malingering are raised as well. In severe cases the functional impairments caused by the dystonia can result in early retirement from work, thus threatening the social status of the patient.

➤ What forms of social help can be offered to patients with dystonia ?

The most effective social help is competent information for members of the family, friends, acquaintances, colleagues at work, the physicians in charge, and medical assistants. Frequently, welfare authorities need to be informed about dystonia and its sequelae.

➤ What is the value of self-help groups ?

As with all other chronic diseases, self-help groups can have a major impact on the psychological and social well-being of patients with dystonia. By increasing public awareness they can contribute to a more rapid diagnosis and thus reduce the often prolonged phase of insecurity for the patient. Public awareness can also help to reduce the lack of understanding experienced by many patients with dystonia. The feelings of isolation and resignation can be markedly reduced by confronting the individual patient with a group of people suffering from the same problems. Exchange of information can improve the patient's knowledge about his or her disorder, as well as about available treatments and treatment facilities. It usually stimulates the patient to take an active role in the treatment of his or her condition and thus helps to stabilise him or her psychologically. Social counselling can provide valuable help to overcome the social problems associated with dystonia.

Cranial Dystonia

➤ What is cranial dystonia ?

The term cranial dystonia describes dystonic hyperactivity in muscles of the head. If it occurs in the eyelid closure muscles it is called blepharospasm. It is one of the most common forms of dystonia. If additional facial muscles are involved the term Meige syndrome is used. Dystonia in jaw muscles is called bruxism. Dystonias of lingual and pharyngeal muscles are less common. If neuroleptic agents are causing cranial dystonia typically perioral, lingual, masticatory, and occasionally pharyngeal muscles are affected. This distribution pattern is known as oroglossomandibular dystonia. Jaw opening dystonia is another rare entity.

➤ What is blepharospasm ?

The term blepharospasm describes dystonic hyperactivity in the orbicularis oculi muscles. Although occasionally one side may be affected more than the other, blepharospasm always involves both orbicularis oculi muscles. In some cases involvement of forehead muscles may be present. Muscle hyperactivity in the frontalis muscle almost always presents compensatory muscle activity rather than primary dystonic involvement. In early stages of the condition symptoms may occur only intermittently. Bright lights, draughts, reading of small print, psychological stress, and physical activity can promote the symptoms, whereas psychological and physical relaxation tend to ameliorate them.

➤ What subtypes of blepharospasm can be distinguished ?

Occasionally blepharospasm may be accompanied by reduced activity of the levator palpebrae muscle in addition to the obligate hyperactivity of the orbicularis oculi muscle. This subtype is known as blepharospasm with eyelid opening apraxia. In some patients, eyelid closure is accompanied by a marked Bell's phenomenon. In rare cases the dystonic hyperactivity is localised predominantly in the palpebral part of the orbicularis oculi muscle. This subtype is called pretarsal blepharospasm. In sensory blepharospasm the patient suffers from marked irritating periocular sensations despite only minor orbicularis oculi hyperactivity.

➤ **What are the differential diagnoses of blepharospasm ?**

All conditions inducing passive eyelid closure, such as myasthenia gravis, paresis of the levator palpebrae muscle and isolated eyelid opening apraxia, must be separated from blepharospasm. Eyelid opening apraxia, often associated with Parkinson's disease and progressive supranuclear palsy, is clinically often difficult to distinguish from blepharospasm. Amimia, as in depressive conditions or Parkinson's disease, can occasionally mimic mild blepharospasm. Mechanical eyelid problems, such as eyelid dehiscences or eyelid oedemas, must also be separated from blepharospasm.

➤ **What examination methods can be used to distinguish between blepharospasm and its differential diagnoses ?**

Electromyography of the orbicularis oculi muscle clearly distinguishes between blepharospasm with a dystonic hyperactivity of the orbicularis oculi muscle and its differential diagnoses lacking this muscle hyperactivity. Needle electromyography of the levator palpebrae muscle can provide additional information. This is especially difficult to perform in patients with impaired reciprocal inhibition between the orbicularis oculi muscle and the levator palpebrae muscle. Unfortunately, this is the main neurophysiological feature of apraxia of eye lid opening.

➤ **What are the possible target muscles for BT therapy for blepharospasm ?**

Figure **17** shows the mimic muscles. The possible target muscles and their recommended therapeutic BT doses are listed in Table **9**. The most important target muscle is the orbicularis oculi muscle. BT is injected between the palpebral part and the orbital part of the muscle. Two injections are usually performed in the lower eyelid. One laterally placed injection is usually sufficient for the upper eyelid. For injections of the upper eyelid it is important not to administer BT into the part of the orbicularis oculi muscle covering the levator palpebrae muscle. All injections in the orbicularis oculi muscle are performed subcutaneously, since – given the thickness of this muscle – attempts at intramuscular injection can easily result in perforation of the muscle with consecutive paresis of external eye muscles. Injections into the corrugator supercilii muscle above the root of the nose, of the procerus muscle at the root of the nose, and the transversal part of the nasalis muscle at the dorsum of the nose may also be performed.

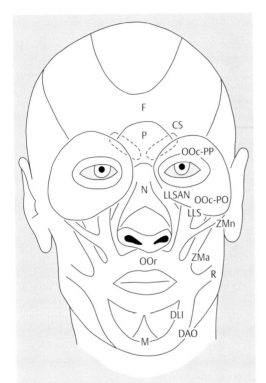

Fig. 17   Mimic muscles.

CS	corrugator supercilii	OOc-PO	orbicularis oculi, orbital part
DAO	depressor anguli oris	OOc-PP	orbicularis oculi, palpebral part
DLI	depressor labii inferioris	OOr	orbicularis oris
F	frontalis	P	procerus
LLS	levator labii superioris	R	risorius
LLSAN	levator labii superioris alaeque nasi	ZMa	zygomaticus major
		ZMn	zygomaticus minor
N	nasalis		

➤ **Should the frontalis muscle be a target muscle of BT therapy for blepharospasm ?**

The frontalis muscle should not be used as a target muscle of BT therapy for blepharospasm since this muscle is an accessory eyelid opener and BT injections would result in weakening of the eyelid opening mechanism.

Table 9 Recommended doses for botulinum toxin therapy of cranial muscles

muscle	function	recommended dose (100 MU-A in 2.5 ml 0.9% NaCl/H$_2$O) [MU-A Botox®]
orbicularis oculi	eyelid closure	18 – 36
procerus	formation of transverse nasal root fold	6 – 12
nasalis (transversal part)	formation of nasal dorsum fold	4 – 8
corrugator supercilii	eyebrow adduction	6 – 12
risorius	corner of mouth abduction	2 – 6
depressor anguli oris	corner of mouth depression	6 – 10
depressor labii inferioris	stabilisation of lower lip	4 – 8
mentalis	formation of chin dimple	6 – 12
levator palpebrae	eyelid opening	16 – 20

MU-A   mouse unit of the mouse bioassay of Allergan Inc

➤ What is the success rate of BT therapy for blepharospasm ?

The success rate of BT therapy for blepharospasm is high. With the exception of the success rate of BT therapy for spasmodic dysphonia, blepharospasm represents the indication for BT therapy with the second highest success rate with practically all patients experiencing substantial benefits. Almost all patients rate the subjective degree of improvement as between 70% and 90%. If involuntary eyelid closures remain at all, their severity is markedly reduced and they usually occur only in special facilitating situations. Complete eyelid closure movements can practically always be eliminated. Figure **18** shows a typical treatment profile of a patient with blepharospasm.

➤ What are the reasons for the high success rate of BT therapy for blepharospasm ?

The high success rate of BT therapy for blepharospasm is due to the properties of the orbicularis oculi muscle. This muscle is an excellent target muscle for BT therapy since its therapeutic window is exceptionally wide, it is easily accessible directly through the skin, and it can clearly be delineated from neighbouring muscles.

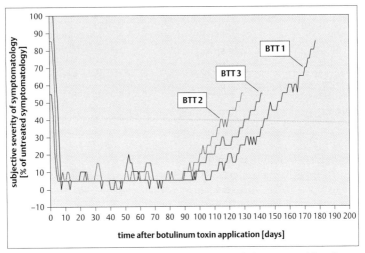

Fig. 18   Treatment profile of a patient with cranial dystonia and botulinum toxin therapy. The profile was reconstructed based on the treatment calendar shown in Fig. **9** (Appendix, p. 128).

BTT 1   botulinum toxin therapy, first application
BTT 2   botulinum toxin therapy, second application
BTT 3   botulinum toxin therapy, third application

➤ What are the factors limiting the success rate of BT therapy for blepharospasm ?

For all differential diagnoses of blepharospasm lacking muscular hyperactivity of the orbicularis oculi muscle BT therapy will not be successful. The success rate will also be limited in subtypes of blepharospasm, such as blepharospasm with an apraxia of eyelid opening component, marked Bell's phenomenon, pretarsal blepharospasm and sensory blepharospasm. Eyelid dehiscences can also limit the success rate.

➤ When is BT therapy for blepharospasm difficult to perform ?

BT therapy for blepharospasm may be difficult to perform in patients with benign eyelid oedema because subcutaneous BT administrations may not reach the orbicularis oculi muscle. In Chinese patients, in whom the skin of the upper eyelid is doubled close to the rim of the eyelid, either as shuang yan pi or dan yan pi, BT administration into the tarsal part of the upper eyelid may also not reach the orbicularis oculi muscle.

➤ **What are the possible side effects
of BT therapy for blepharospasm ?**

All possible side effects of BT therapy for blepharospasm are local side effects. Paresis of the levator palpebrae muscle inducing ptosis can occur occasionally. Its frequency should be less than 5% of the injection series and its duration is usually limited to two weeks. BT therapy induced ptosis is almost always partial. Complete ptosis is a very rare complication. Double vision due to paresis of external eye muscles is another possible side effect. Most often it is caused by BT diffusion into the rectus lateralis muscle. In most cases the double vision is noticed only in extreme gaze positions. A discrete weakening of the corner of the mouth may arise in individual cases, but this usually has no functional significance. Haematomas at the injection site cannot always be avoided, but their extent can be reduced by adequate compression of the injection site. Persisting pain or tissue irritations have not been observed.

➤ **What are the factors facilitating side effects
of BT therapy for blepharospasm ?**

Side effects of BT therapy for blepharospasm are facilitated by loose consistency of the tarsal and orbital connective tissues as often seen in the elderly. It is thought that the loose consistency can result in more wide-spread diffusion of BT and of haematomas. It seems that occurrence of ptosis and double vision are facilitated by exophthalmic conditions.

➤ **What other treatments are available
when BT therapy for blepharospasm fails ?**

In patients with blepharospasm selective peripheral denervation or dissections of the orbicularis oculi muscle can be performed. Medical treatment for dystonia may be tried, but is usually of limited benefit. In patients with apraxia of eyelid opening a subcutaneous eyelid suspension can be applied to fix the upper eyelid to the forehead muscles. In patients with a combination of eyelid opening apraxia and blepharospasm suspension operations and BT therapy can be combined. In those patients spectacle frames with specially attached spring devices to fix the upper lids may also be tried. In patients with eyelid dehiscences lifting operations are helpful.

➤ **What are the possible problems associated
with surgical treatment of blepharospasm?**

With selective peripheral denervation operations re-innervation processes occur in a large proportion of the patients within a few months after the operation thus antagonising the benefit of the procedure. Primary re-operations are frequently necessary to achieve satisfactory results. Unpleasant, long-lasting pain in the operation region can also occur. Suspension operations and eyelid lifting operations are not helpful as long as the blepharospasm continues since the forces released by the blepharospasm quickly antagonise their effect.

➤ **What is Meige syndrome?**

The term Meige syndrome describes dystonic hyperactivity affecting not only the periocular muscles but also other cranial muscles. These are most frequently perioral muscles and lingual muscles. However, jaw muscles and pharyngeal muscles may also be affected.

➤ **What are the possible target muscles
for BT therapy for Meige syndrome?**

Figure **17** (p. 54) shows the mimic muscles. The possible target muscles and their recommended therapeutic BT doses are listed in Table **9** (p. 55). In addition to the target muscles of BT therapy for blepharospasm, lower facial muscles can also be used in patients with Meige syndrome. Thus, in the region of the corner of the mouth the risorius muscle, the depressor anguli oris muscle, and the depressor labii inferioris muscle can be injected. In the chin region the mentalis muscle is a possible target muscle.

➤ **What are the problems associated
with BT therapy for lower facial muscles?**

Target muscles of the lower face have very narrow therapeutic windows. Thus, BT injections into these target muscles can easily induce functional and cosmetic impairments. BT dosing in these target muscles must therefore be calculated carefully.

➤ **Which muscles should be avoided
in BT therapy for Meige syndrome ?**

All muscles lifting the corner of the mouth, such as the levator labii superioris muscle, the levator angulis oris muscle, and the zygomatic
muscles should not be used as target muscles. These muscles have extremely narrow therapeutic windows, so that functional and cosmetic
impairments will frequently result. BT injections into the orbicularis oris muscle in the upper lip can induce dysaesthesias usually described by
the patient as a disturbing swelling or tingling sensation. This muscle
should therefore also be avoided.

➤ **What is the success rate of BT therapy for Meige syndrome ?**

For periocular muscles the success rate of BT therapy for Meige syndrome is identical to the success rate of BT therapy for blepharospasm.
BT injection in additional muscles is rather difficult because of their exceptionally narrow therapeutic windows. Even several attempts to optimise the BT dose usually induce only partial improvement of the condition.

➤ **What are the possible side effects
of BT therapy for Meige syndrome ?**

In addition to the possible side effects of BT therapy for blepharospasm,
BT injections into lower facial muscles can induce functional impairment with instabilities of the lower lips and accidental bite injuries during eating. Additionally, cosmetic impairment due to paresis of the ab-
ductors of the corner of the mouth can occur.

➤ **What is bruxism ?**

The term bruxism describes dystonic hyperactivity in the jaw muscles.
This muscle hyperactivity may be limited to individual jaw muscles, but
usually it involves all jaw muscles. The severity of bruxism varies greatly. In mild cases the symptomatology only occurs in situations of psychological stress, such as examinations or marital crises. It is still not
known whether these forms represent dystonias. They do not induce
functional impairment and sequelae are not to be expected. In severe
cases sensations of tension in the jaw muscles are reported and the
dental status and the mandibular joints may be impaired. Very severe
bruxism, not infrequently caused by mid brain lesions, is usually ac-

companied by additional craniocervical dystonia and is almost inevitably followed by severe functional impairment and often massive damage to the dental status and the mandibular joints. In these cases pain, usually severe and intense, results not only from muscular overuse but also from secondary damage.

➤ When should bruxism be treated with BT ?

For cases of bruxism with minor symptomatology BT therapy is not indicated. In these cases psychotherapeutical intervention and, at the most, mild transient psychopharmacotherapy should be used. In moderately severe cases, dental protection should be worn at night additionally. Should these interventions fail, a trial of BT therapy may be considered to break the vicious circle. Severe cases of bruxism with intense pain symptoms, marked functional impairment or with development of secondary damage are a clear indication of BT therapy.

➤ What are the possible target muscles for BT therapy for bruxism ?

The function of the jaw muscles are listed in Table **10.** The possible target muscles and their recommended therapeutic BT doses are listed in Table **11.** Usually bilateral BT administration into the masseter muscles is sufficient. Additional BT injection into the temporalis muscles may be tried in more severe cases. In massive bruxism, especially in cases with jaw protrusion, additional BT administration in the pterygoideus muscles becomes necessary.

➤ How can the pterygoideus muscles be accessed ?

The pterygoideus muscles can be accessed through the outer oral cavity or – under wide jaw opening – transcutaneously through the mandibular notch.

➤ What is the success rate of BT therapy for bruxism ?

Usually, pain responds particularly well to BT therapy for bruxism. In most cases pain will almost completely be eliminated. In severe cases functional impairment can be reduced so that, for example, fitting of dentures will become possible. BT therapy may prevent the progression of secondary damage due to bruxism although existing damage will not be diminished.

Table 10 Jaw muscle functions under physiological conditions

function	muscle	estimated degree of involvement
jaw closing	temporalis	1
	masseter	2
	pterygoideus medialis	3
jaw opening	suprahyoidal muscles	1
	digastricus	2
	pterygoideus lateralis	3
	neck extensors	4
jaw protrusion	pterygoideus lateralis	1
	pterygoideus medialis	2
jaw lateralisation	pterygoideus medialis	1

Table 11 Recommended doses for botulinum toxin therapy of bruxism

muscle	function	recommended dose (100 MU-A in 2.5 ml 0.9% NaCl/H_2O) [MU-A Botox®]
temporalis	jaw closing	40 – 80
masseter	jaw closing	40 – 80
pterygoidei	jaw closing jaw protrusion jaw lateralisation	20 – 40

MU-A   mouse unit of the mouse bioassay of Allergan Inc

➤ **What are the possible side effects of BT therapy for bruxism** ?

Potential side effects of BT therapy for bruxism are few and rare. Although paresis of masticatory muscle is obligatory, this weakness is often not noticed. Occasionally, BT induced paresis may present as premature fatigue during intensive chewing. Changes of the eating habits are not to be expected.

➤ **What is the experience with BT therapy
   for jaw opening dystonia ?**

Experience with BT therapy for jaw opening dystonia is limited. Table
10 lists the muscles responsible for jaw opening. The main problem
with jaw opening dystonia is that the suprahyoidal muscles as the major jaw openers are hardly suitable for BT injection because of possible
paretic side effects in the lingual muscles. Clinical experience shows
that jaw closing muscles are often activated in jaw opening dystonia,
especially with extreme jaw opening movements. BT injections into
these muscles is therefore sometimes helpful, especially for pain reduction and prevention of secondary temporomandibular joint damage.
The lateral pterygoid muscle can elegantly be reached transcutaneously
through the incissura mundibulae when the jaw is opened.

➤ **What is the experience with BT therapy for lingual dystonia ?**

Experience with BT therapy for lingual dystonia is limited. Since the lingual muscles have a very narrow therapeutic window, severe functional
impairment, such as swallowing or articulation problems, is common.
BT injections into lingual muscles should therefore be avoided.

Cervical Dystonia

➤ **What is torticollis ?**

The term torticollis describes sustained abnormal positioning of the
neck. It is a descriptive term not implying any specific aetiology.

➤ **What are the conditions causing torticollis ?**

Distorted neck positioning or torticollis can be caused by a number of
different conditions. In neurogenic torticollis, cervical dystonia or spasmodic torticollis caused by muscle hyperactivity and apraxic conditions
or impairment of the body image caused by central nervous system
dysfunction can be distinguished. A number of ophthalmological, orthopaedic and vestibular disorders can induce abnormal neck posture
as well. Occasionally, torticollis may be caused by traumatic shortening
of the sternocleidomastoid muscle at birth. Psychogenic torticollis is
equally rare. In BT therapy for cervical dystonia it is important to be
aware of the spectrum of conditions causing torticollis, since only cervical dystonia will respond to BT therapy.

➤ **What is cervical dystonia ?**

The term cervical dystonia describes dystonic hyperactivity in neck muscles producing abnormal neck positions.

➤ **How can cervical dystonia be classified with regard to the plane of head rotation ?**

Head rotation in a horizontal plane is called torticollis, head rotation in a frontal plane is referred to as laterocollis and head rotation in a sagittal plane is named antecollis or retrocollis. In most patients there is a combination of several of these elements. If the term cervical dystonia is used as a general description, the terms torticollis, laterocollis, retrocollis, and antecollis can be used to describe the individual elements of the head rotation. The term torticollis spasticus is misleading, since torticollis is a dystonic condition and not a spastic one.

➤ **How can cervical dystonia be documented ?**

Documentation of cervical dystonia can be helpful for evaluation of the therapeutic effect of BT therapy, for documentation of fluctuations and for identification of facilitating factors. This documentation can be performed with clinical rating scales. Table **12** shows a clinical rating scale which is easy to use. Table **6** (Appendix, p. 130) gives a video protocol for complete documentation of the clinical symptomatology in cervical dystonia. Figure **19** shows an instrument for measuring the angles of head and neck deviation.

➤ **Is there a standardised BT therapy for cervical dystonia ?**

There is no standardised BT therapy for cervical dystonia. BT therapy for cervical dystonia is always highly individualised for each particular patient since the extent and localisation of the dystonic muscle hyperactivity within the numerous neck muscles are subject to broad interindividual variations.

➤ **What is the main objective for planning BT therapy for cervical dystonia ?**

Planning of BT therapy for cervical dystonia has two main objectives. Firstly, the dystonic muscles have to be identified. Secondly, the extent of their dystonic involvement must be established. This information al-

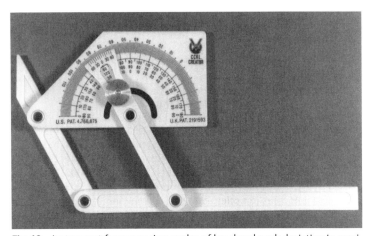

Fig. 19   Instrument for measuring angles of head and neck deviation in cervical dystonia.

Table 12   Cervical dystonia rating scale according to Tsui (Tsui JKC, Eisen A, Stoessl AJ, Calne S, Calne DB. Double-blind study of botulinum toxin in spasmodic torticollis. Lancet 1986 II: 245 – 247)

section	item	score
A	amplitude of sustained movements	
	rotation: 0 = absent, 1 = $<15^0$, 2 = $15-30^0$, 3 = $>30^0$	0 1 2 3
	tilt: $\quad$ 0 = absent, 1 = $<15^0$, 2 = $15-30^0$, 3 = $>30^0$	0 1 2 3
	antecollis/retrocollis:	0 1 2 3
	$\quad$ 0 = absent, 1 = mild, 2 = moderate, 3 = severe	A =
	score A = rotation + tilt + antecollis/retrocollis	
B	duration of sustained movements	
	1 = intermittent	1 2
	2 = constant	B =
C	shoulder elevation	
	0 = absent	0 1 2 3
	1 = mild and intermittent	C =
	2 = mild and constant or severe and intermittent	
	3 = severe and constant	
D	tremor	
	severity: 0 = absent, 1 = mild, 2 = severe	0 1 2
	duration: 0 = absent, 1 = occasional, 2 = continuous	0 1 2
	score D = severity X duration	D =
	total score = $(A \times B) + C + D$ =	

lows the BT dose to be set as high as necessary and as low as possible in order to ensure both a sufficient therapeutic effect as well as avoidance of side effects. Additionally, muscles with compensatory activity need to be identified and have to be spared from BT administration.

➤ **How can cervical dystonia be evaluated with respect to planning of BT therapy ?**

A careful clinical examination should document the direction and the extent of the head position at rest, under usual physical activity and under provoking conditions. Table **13** gives an overview of the functions of the main neck muscles under physiological conditions. This information provides some preliminary insight into the dystonic involvement of the various neck muscles. Preventive head posturing, sometimes used by patients to avoid triggering of dystonia, needs to be identified and distinguished from dystonic positioning. Passive neck movements should be tested to assess secondary damage due to cervical dystonia. Table **14** shows the range of passive neck mobility under physiological conditions. Secondary damage will not respond to BT therapy and will therefore limit its outcome. An exact case history helps to understand the severity of the condition with all its fluctuations as well as the individual impairment caused by it. This information helps to distinguish dystonic complaints requiring treatment from those which do not. Electromyographic examinations should be carried out to identify dystonic muscles and to determine the extent of their dystonic involvement. They can also be helpful in identification of compensatory muscle activity. Localisation of focal pain, especially in muscles of the side and the back of the neck, provides additional clues as to the identification of more severely affected dystonic muscles.

➤ **Why is planning of BT therapy for cervical dystonia solely guided by clinical observations problematic ?**

Dystonic co-contractions in antagonistic muscles occur frequently and cannot be detected by clinical evaluation of the head position alone. Without electromyography, identification of dystonic involvement of deep neck muscles and of compensatory muscle activity is difficult. Quantification of dystonic involvement can only be performed with electromyography.

Table 13 Neck muscle function under physiological conditions

function	muscle	estimated degree of involvement
head and neck flexion	hyoid muscles	1
	longus colli	2
	longus capitis	3
	rectus capitis anterior	4
head and neck extension	semispinalis capitis	1
	trapezius, cervical part	2
	splenius capitis	3
	longissimus capitis	4
	rectus capitis posterior major	5
	rectus capitis posterior minor	5
head and neck rotation	sternocleidomastoideus	1
	splenius capitis	2
	trapezius, cervical part	3
	longissimus capitis	4
	obliquus capitis inferior	5
	rectus capitis posterior major	5
	rectus capitis posterior minor	5
head and neck lateral flexion	sternocleidomastoideus	1
	scalenus anterior	2
	scalenus medius	2
	scalenus posterior	2
	levator scapulae	3
	splenius capitis	4
	trapezius, cervical part	5
	semispinalis	6
	longissimus capitis	7
	longissimus cervicis	7
	multifidus	8
	obliquus capitis inferior	9
	obliquus capitis superior	9
	rectus capitis posterior major	9
head and neck protrusion	sternocleidomastoideus	1
head and neck retrusion	splenius capitis	1
	levator scapulae	2

Table 14 Normal passive neck mobility

plane	head movement	degree of mobility	remarks
sagittal	extension flexion	40° 70°	one third of head movement in upper and lower head joint two thirds of head movement in neck joints
sagittal	protrusion retrusion	approx. 5 cm approx. 5 cm	
frontal	lateral flexion	45°	
transversal	rotation	90°	one third of head movement in upper and lower head joint two thirds of head movement in neck joints

➤ **How can electromyographic evaluation of cervical dystonia be performed ?**

Electromyographic evaluation of cervical dystonia tries to identify and to quantify dystonic neck muscle involvement. For this 2 channel needle recordings of the major neck muscle groups, the trapezius/semispinalis muscles, the splenius capitis muscles, the levator scapulae muscles, the scalenii muscles and the sternocleidomastoid muscles, are performed. To quantify their dystonic involvement the ratio between the electromyographic activity under maximal voluntary activation and under spontaneous conditions are calculated. These dystonia ratios can be displayed as shown in Figure **20.** Passive head movements and observations of the onset pattern of dystonic muscle hyperactivity help to distinguish preventive head positioning and compensatory muscle activity.

➤ **What are the possible target muscles for BT therapy for cervical dystonia ?**

Figures **21** to **23** show the neck muscles. The possible target muscles and their recommended therapeutic BT doses are listed in Table **15.** The target muscle selection is based exclusively on the patient's individual symptomatology.

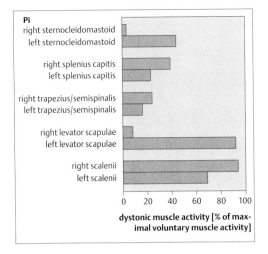

Fig. 20 a Dystonia ratios in a patient with cervical dystonia. The dystonia ratio is the ratio between the needle electromyographic activity in a test muscle under maximal voluntary activation and under spontaneous conditions.

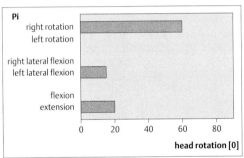

b Corresponding head position.

rSCM	right sternocleidomastoid	rScal	right scalenii
lSCM	left sternocleidomastoid	lScal	left scalenii
rSC	right splenius capitis	rR	right rotation
lSC	left splenius capitis	lR	left rotation
rT/SS	right trapezius/semispinalis	rLF	right lateral flexion
lT/SS	left trapezius/semispinalis	lLF	left lateral flexion
rLS	right levator scapulae	F	flexion
lLS	left levator scapulae	E	extension

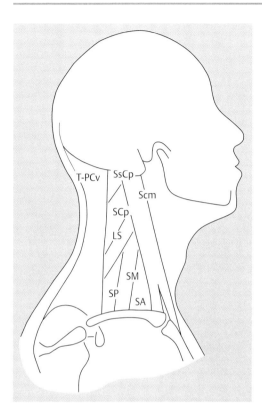

Fig. 21 Neck muscles; lateral view.

LS	levator scapulae	SM	scalenus medius
SA	scalenus anterior	SP	scalenus posterior
Scm	sternocleidomastoideus	SsCp	semispinalis capitis
SCp	splenius capitis	T-PCv	trapezius, cervical part

➤ **How can BT injections into the
sternocleidomastoid muscle be optimised?**

For BT injections into the sternocleidomastoid muscle it is essential to avoid penetration of the muscle and BT injection into the underlying muscles involved in the generation of swallowing. For this the manipulation shown in Figure **24** can be helpful.

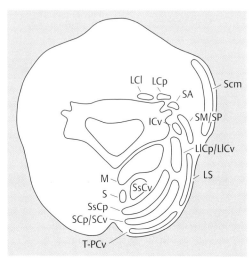

Fig. 22 Neck muscles; transverse section at level C5.

ICv	iliocostalis cervicis	Scm	sternocleidomastoideus
LCl	longus colli	SCp/SCv	splenius capitis/splenius cervicis
LCp	longus capitis		
LS	levator scapulae	SM/SP	scalenus medius/scalenus posterior
LlCp/LlCv	longissimus capitis/ longissimus cervicis		
		SsCp	semispinalis capitis
M	multifidus	SsCv	semispinalis cervicis
S	spinalis	T-PCv	trapezius, cervical part
SA	scalenus anterior		

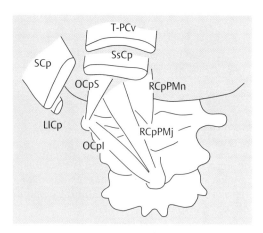

Fig. 23 Short neck muscles.

Table 15 Recommended doses for botulinum toxin therapy of cervical muscles

muscle	function	recommended dose (100 MU-A in 2.5 ml 0.9% NaCl/H$_2$O) [MU-A Botox®]
sternocleidomastoid	contralateral horizontal head rotation sagittal head flexion ipsilateral frontal head flexion head protrusion	20 – 80
splenius capitis	ipsilateral horizontal head rotation sagittal head extension ipsilateral frontal head flexion head retrusion	20 – 60
scalenus anterior	frontal head flexion	20 – 60
scalenus medius	frontal head flexion	20 – 60
scalenus posterior	frontal head flexion	20 – 60
levator scapulae	ipsilateral frontal head flexion shoulder elevation ipsilateral horizontal head rotation	20 – 60
trapezius, cervical part, and semispinalis	sagittal head extension ipsilateral horizontal head rotation ipsilateral frontal head flexion	20 – 60
trapezius, horizontal part	shoulder elevation frontal head flexion	40 – 80

MU-A   mouse unit of the mouse bioassay of Allergan Inc

◀ **Fig. 23** *Abbreviations*

LlCp	longissimus capitis	RCpPMn	rectus capitis posterior minor
OCpI	obliquus capitis inferior	SCp	splenius capitis
OCpS	obliquus capitis superior	SsCp	semispinalis capitis
RCpPMj	rectus capitis posterior major	T-PCv	trapezius, cervical part

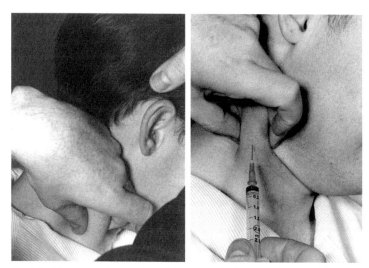

Fig. 24 Manoeuvre for fixation of the sternocleidomastoid muscle for botulinum toxin injections. **a** The patient's head is manipulated into a position in which the sternocleidomastoid muscle becomes maximally prominent. The sternocleidomastoid muscle is then held firmly with the fingers reaching behind the muscle. **b** The botulinum toxin injections are performed.

➤ **What is the success rate of BT therapy for cervical dystonia ?**

The success rate of BT therapy for cervical dystonia is high. All patients will experience at least some degree of improvement of their symptomatology. Practically all patients will estimate the degree of their improvement to be in the range of 70 to 90%. Usually, head control will be improved to the extent that the underlying cervical dystonia will not be noticed by an untrained observer under most conditions. However, in facilitating situations, such as physical exercise or psychological stress, involuntary movements may be noticed. These isolated movements, however, are substantially less severe and less frequent than before. If pain is present its improvement is usually even better than the improvement of involuntary movements. Practically all patients report an improvement of their pain symptoms by about 80 to 100%. Figure **25** shows a typical treatment profile for a patient with cervical dystonia.

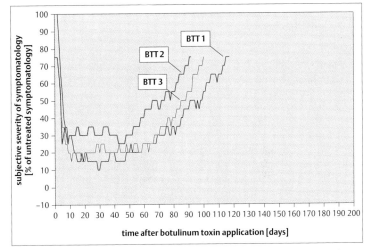

Fig. 25 Treatment profile of a patient with cervical dystonia and botulinum toxin therapy. The profile was reconstructed based on the treatment calendar shown in Fig. **9** (Appendix, p. 128).

BTT 1   botulinum toxin therapy, first application
BTT 2   botulinum toxin therapy, second application
BTT 3   botulinum toxin therapy, third application

➤ **Can physiotherapy improve the outcome
of BT therapy for cervical dystonia ?**

Physiotherapy in addition to BT therapy can be useful to mobilise muscle contractures and to increase passive neck mobility. Physiotherapy can also help to re-adjust impaired postural head reflexes, especially in patients with long-standing conditions. Lack of re-adjustment training should not be underestimated as a possible cause for partial primary BT therapy failure in cervical dystonia.

➤ **Are there differences in the success rates of BT therapy
in patients with tonic, clonic and tremolous cervical dystonia ?**

From all experience available so far, the success rates of BT therapy are not significantly different for these forms of cervical dystonia, although we believe that tremolous forms of cervical dystonia may possibly respond less favourably than other forms.

➤ **What subtypes of cervical dystonia are difficult to treat with BT therapy ?**

Antecollis is a subtype of cervical dystonia which is usually difficult to treat with BT therapy. It can exist in two different forms. The first form is a pure head flexion caused by bilateral contraction of the sternoclei- domastoid muscles. This form responds well to BT therapy, although careful dosing is advised to avoid swallowing problems more common after bilateral sternocleidomastoid injections. The second form involves a head protrusion, a combination of neck flexion and head extension. This form is caused by contractions of prevertebral neck flexors and head extensors. Since BT injection into prevertebral neck flexors are technically difficult to perform, the therapeutic outcome in these pa- tients is usually unsatisfactory. Careful BT administration into the neck extensors, however, may sometimes be of limited benefit.

➤ **What are the differential diagnoses of cervical dystonia unresponsive to BT therapy ?**

BT does not exhibit therapeutic action on all conditions not caused by muscle hyperactivity, such as apraxic conditions, impairment of the body image and all non-neurogenic forms of torticollis.

➤ **When is BT therapy for cervical dystonia difficult to perform ?**

BT therapy for cervical dystonia may be difficult to perform in patients with short necks, thick skin and thick subcutaneous tissue complicating anatomical orientation.

➤ **What are the possible side effects of BT therapy for cervical dystonia ?**

BT therapy for cervical dystonia can cause functional impairment of the target muscle, clinically manifesting as reduced head control. Weaken- ing of muscles adjacent to the target muscles due to BT diffusion can in- duce dysphagia. Occasionally patients may report of dry mouth. This can probably be attributed to impairment of the cholinergic innervation of the salivary glands.

➤ **What is the extent of reduced head control
after BT therapy for cervical dystonia ?**

The extent of reduced head control after BT therapy is usually noticed only in particular situations, such as looking up when bending forwards, rising from supine positions and intensive physical exercise.

➤ **What is the frequency of reduced head control
after BT therapy for cervical dystonia ?**

Since the severity of side effects is not stated in most studies, reports on their frequency are difficult to interpret. In our experience, a reduction of head control with changes in daily life occurs in less than 5 % of the patients.

➤ **What is the extent of dysphagia
after BT therapy for cervical dystonia ?**

In most cases of dysphagia patients will only become aware of the swallowing process. In more severe cases, the patients may report increased number of swallowing attempts accompanied by a bolus sensation in the throat. Changes in food intake, either concerning the consistency or the amount of food, are rare. Aspirations have been reported in the literature on a few occasions, but when they do occur they should be dealt with appropriately by nasogastric tube and antibiosis.

➤ **What is the frequency of dysphagia
after BT therapy for cervical dystonia ?**

Again, since the severity of dysphagia is not mentioned in most studies, figures on the frequency of dysphagia are difficult to interpret. According to our experience, mild dysphagia is relatively common and may be experienced by as many as one third of the patients. More severe dysphagia causing changes in eating habits occurs in certainly less than 5 % of the patients.

➤ **What are the causes of dysphagia
after BT therapy for cervical dystonia ?**

The cause of dysphagia has not been finally elucidated. On one hand, dysphagia may arise from BT diffusion into neighbouring swallowing muscles. In this way, BT injections into the sternocleidomastoid muscle close to its origin would be particularly prone to produce dysphagia. On the other hand, dysphagia could arise from systemic BT spread. Interestingly, swallowing is one of the first functions to be disturbed in botulism, indicating a low reserve strength of these muscles. Systemic distribution after use of high BT doses can explain dysphagia when BT is administered to a body region distant from the neck.

➤ **What is the duration of side effects of BT therapy for cervical dystonia ?**

Dysphagia usually occurs about 10 days after the BT injection and then lasts for about 10 days. Reduced head control usually also starts about 10 days after BT injection, but then persists somewhat longer than the dysphagia.

➤ **How can the side effects of BT therapy for cervical dystonia be avoided ?**

Reduction of head control can be avoided by reducing the BT dose injected into the head extensors or head flexors. At least after a few BT injections series, it should be possible to achieve sufficient strength and duration of the therapeutic BT effect without reduced head control. Only rarely is reduced head control induced by excessive weakening of lateral neck muscles. Dysphagia can be avoided by reducing the BT dose injected into the sternocleidomastoid muscles. It may also be possible to reduce dysphagia by BT administration into the distal part of the sternocleidomastoid muscle, i.e., the part of the muscle close to the cranium. In some patients slight dysphagia cannot always be avoided even after numerous attempts to optimise BT dosages.

➤ **What other treatments are available when BT therapy for cervical dystonia fails ?**

If BT therapy for cervical dystonia fails drug treatment should be tried next. If this drug treatment is also unsuccessful, the next therapeutic option is the Bertrand operation, classically a combination of resection of the dorsal branches of the anterior roots (ramisectomy), peripheral denervation and dissection of the contralateral sternocleidomastoid muscle and ipsilateral short neck muscles. Stereotactic interventions should be reserved for the most severe forms of cervical dystonia. Epidural spinal electrostimulation has been tried, but has very uncertain efficacy and risks of infection and electrode breakage are high.

Pharyngolaryngeal Dystonia

➤ **What forms of pharyngolaryngeal dystonia
can be distinguished ?**

By far the most frequent form of pharyngolaryngeal dystonia is spasmodic dysphonia. Markedly less common is pharyngeal dystonia, which mostly occurs in combination with cranial dystonia. Equally rare are combinations of pharyngeal dystonia and laryngeal dystonia. Another very rare form of laryngeal dystonia is laryngeal spasmodic dyspnea.

➤ **Can pharyngolaryngeal dystonia be the initial symptom
of a spreading dystonic symptomatology ?**

Although pharyngolaryngeal dystonia can occur in the context of a wide-spread dystonia, pharyngolaryngeal dystonia is not the initial localisation of spreading dystonia.

➤ **What is spasmodic dysphonia ?**

The term spasmodic dysphonia describes dystonic hyperactivity in larynx muscles causing impaired phonation. Since the dystonic muscle hyperactivity occurs almost exclusively during speech and not spontaneously, spasmodic dysphonia is a typical action-induced dystonia. Phonations not associated with speech, such as singing, are frequently not impaired. In cases of spasmodic dysphonia, the patients complain of a strained and strangled voice that fails intermittently. The flow of speech is slow and hesitant. As with other forms of dystonia, symptoms usually become more pronounced under psychological and physical stress. Supraglottic and pharyngeal involvement can occur occasionally. Stridor with dyspnea is not a feature of spasmodic dysphonia, although patients may have reduced phonatory air because of the hesitant flow of speech.

➤ **What forms of spasmodic dysphonia can be distinguished ?**

By far the most frequent form of spasmodic dysphonia is the adductor form, in which the dystonic muscle hyperactivity occurs in the vocal cord adductor, the cricothyroid muscle, the lateral cricoarytenoid muscle, and the interarytenoid muscle. Much less frequent is the abductor form, in which the dystonic muscle hyperactivity occurs in the vocal cord abductor and the posterior cricoarytenoid muscle. This form is characterised by a typical hypophonia. Mixtures of the adductor and abductor forms exist, but are extremely rare.

➤ How can spasmodic dysphonia be documented?

Spasmodic dysphonia can be documented by asking the patient to read a standard passage as shown in Table **16** (Appendix, p. 137). Table **17** (Appendix, p. 137) gives an assessment protocol unmarking the mayor aspects of spasmodic dysphonia. A rating scale for spasmodic dysphonia is presented in Table **18** (Appendix, p. 138).

➤ What is spasmodic laryngeal dyspnoea?

The term spasmodic laryngeal dyspnoea is used to describe spontaneously occurring or respiration-induced muscle hyperactivity of laryngeal muscles. This condition is very rare and may influence both glottic and supraglottic muscles.

➤ How is BT therapy for pharyngolaryngeal dystonia performed?

Usually, BT therapy for pharyngolaryngeal dystonia is performed as an out-patient procedure. After thorough anaesthesia of the pharyngolaryngeal mucosa, the target muscles are inspected laryngoscopically. BT administration is performed by using a butterfly cannula with a flexible tube and held by a specially designed instrument, which is shown in Figure **26.** The advantage of this perioral administration technique is optimal control of the injection site both for pharyngeal and for laryngeal BT injections. In anatomically unfavourable conditions pharyngolaryngeal BT therapy may be performed under general anaesthesia. Then, however, a short hospitalisation becomes necessary. As an alternative to the perioral approach, a transcutaneous access may be used for BT therapy for adductor forms of spasmodic dysphonia. In this case, a combined EMG injection cannula is advanced through the cricothyroid membrane into the target muscle. Exact positioning of the injection cannula is controlled by a simultaneous EMG recording of the target muscle. The combined EMG-injection cannula is shown in Figure **27.**

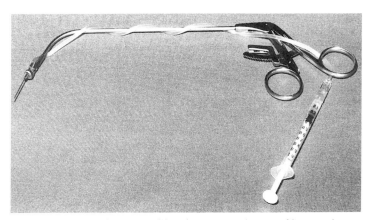

Fig. 26   Instrument for transoral botulinum toxin therapy of laryngopharyngeal dystonia.

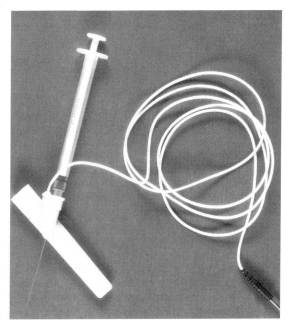

Fig. 27
Combined EMG-injection cannula (Allergan Inc). By means of the combined EMG-injection cannula botulinum toxin can be injected into the target muscle under continuous electromyographic control.

➤ **What are the advantages and the disadvantages of the transcutaneous approach for BT therapy for spasmodic dysphonia ?**

The transcutaneous approach is simple, quick, less unpleasant for the patient and can be carried out with equipment easily available. Its disadvantage, however, is that the dystonic pharyngolaryngeal movements cannot be inspected so that diagnostic misinterpretations are possible. In particular, involvement of non-laryngeal muscles cannot be diagnosed by this method. In our opinion, the perioral approach in BT therapy for pharyngolaryneal dystonia with visualisation of the affected muscles is the superior procedure.

➤ **What are the possible target muscles for BT therapy for pharyngolaryngeal dystonia ?**

The possible target muscles and their recommended therapeutic BT doses are listed in Table **19.** In adductor forms of spasmodic dysphonia, BT is administered into the thyreoarytenoid or vocalis muscle. Injections may be made on both sides or on one side alone. It appears that unilateral injections seem to produce less side effects than bilateral injections. In abductor forms of spasmodic dysphonia, BT is administered into the posterior cricoarytenoid muscle unilaterally in order to avoid dyspnoea. In BT therapy for laryngeal spasmodic dyspnoea and pharyngeal dystonia the selection of the target muscle depends on the respective localisation of the dystonic muscle hyperactivity.

Table 19 Recommended doses for botulinum toxin therapy of laryngeal muscles

muscle	function	recommended dose (100 MU-A in 2.5 ml 0.9 % NaCl/H$_2$O) [MU-A Botox®]
thyreoarytenoid (vocalis)	vocal cord adduction vocal cord tension	unilateral injection: 2.5 – 10 bilateral injection: 1.25 – 5
posterior cricoarytenoid	vocal cord abduction	unilateral injection: 2.5 – 10

MU-A   mouse unit of the mouse bioassay of Allergan Inc

➤ **What BT doses should be used
in BT therapy for spasmodic dysphonia ?**

In BT therapy for spasmodic dysphonia a wide range of dosages has been used. For adductor forms and unilateral administration the reported doses range from 0.625 to 25 mouse units Botox®. In BT therapy for adductor forms unilateral injection of 2.5 to 10 mouse units Botox® or bilateral injection of 1.25 to 5 mouse units Botox® should be adequate. In BT therapy for abductor forms unilateral BT administration should be used exclusively.

➤ **What is the success rate of BT therapy for spasmodic dysphonia ?**

For the patient and for the physician, BT therapy for spasmodic dysphonia represents a very satisfying indication. Practically all patients benefit from BT therapy and the degree of improvement is astonishing. In many cases almost normal speech patterns can be regained. In patients with abductor forms the treatment results are less favourable. But even here most patients notice an improvement of their condition. In BT therapy for spasmodic dysphonia, the therapeutic effect usually begins after 2 to 3 days, reaches its maximum after about 4 to 5 days and then lasts for 2 to 9 months with an average duration of about 4 months.

➤ **What are the possible side effects
of BT therapy for spasmodic dysphonia ?**

BT therapy for spasmodic dysphonia can produce difficulties with swallowing liquids or solid food. It can also induce weakness of coughing and some pain at the injection side. In treatment of adductor forms, hoarseness, breathiness of voice, and hypophonia can occur. Reports on the frequency of these side effects are contradictory. Most of the patients will have to expect mild forms of hoarseness and hypophonia for a period of about one to three weeks after treatment. However, given the dramatic improvement after treatment, patients readily accept these temporary side effects. Serious side effects are not to be expected after BT therapy of adductor forms. In treatment of abductor forms dyspnoea may occur. For this reason BT therapies for abductor forms should only be carried by qualified personnel in selected institutions.

➤ **What is the experience with BT therapy for pharyngeal dystonia and laryngeal spasmodic dyspnea ?**

Only few reports have been published on BT therapy for pharyngeal dystonia and spasmodic laryngeal dyspnea. For these indications initiation of BT therapy depends on the severity of the impairment caused by the condition. The treatment results for these indications depend on the symptomatology treated.

Limb Dystonia

➤ **What is limb dystonia ?**

The term limb dystonia describes dystonic hyperactivity in muscles of the arms or the legs.

➤ **What forms of limb dystonia can be distinguished ?**

Limb dystonia can be divided into action-induced and non-action-induced forms. Action-induced forms occur only during certain activities which can sometimes be highly specific. Non-action-induced forms are not associated with specific activities, although they may be increased by specific and unspecific activities.

➤ **What forms of action-induced limb dystonia can be distinguished ?**

Action-induced limb dystonia occurs almost exclusively in the upper extremities with writer's cramp being the most common form. Apart from writing there are a number of other highly specific and sometimes peculiar activities that trigger dystonia, such as playing musical instruments or performing sports. Many of these rare conditions are induced by frequently performed activities suggesting that overuse may be a causal factor for their occurrence. Claims of high prevalence of writer's cramp amongst clerical staff at the end of last century may be interpreted in this context. Action-induced limb dystonia may also be triggered by emotion-charged activities. A combination of overuse and emotional involvement, as seen in professional musicians or professional athletes, could be especially dangerous for development of limb dystonia. For these forms of action-induced dystonia the term occupational cramps has been coined.

In action-induced limb dystonia functional impairment is usually the main complaint. Depending on the triggering activity, the patient's degree of disability varies greatly. Pain symptoms are usually rare, since the total duration of occurrence of dystonic muscle hyperactivity is limited.

➤ **What is writer's cramp ?**

The term writer's cramp describes dystonic hyperactivity of forearm muscles and occasionally also proximal arm muscles, of shoulder muscles and small hand muscles which are triggered by writing movements. Initially, only flowing hand-writing is a trigger. Later in the course of the disease, dystonia can also be triggered by writing printed characters, by drawing and even by pure contact with writing utensils. Finally, other motor activities can be triggers. The occurrence of dystonic muscle hyperactivity leads to functional impairment, which is often compensated over a long period of time by various sensory or motor tricks. Abnormal elbow and shoulder positions can be voluntarily used to suppress the occurrence of the dystonic muscle hyperactivity. Pain can occur in advanced stages of the disease and patients who write frequently tend to view pain increasingly as their major problem.

➤ **What forms of non-action-induced limb dystonia can be distinguished ?**

Non-action-induced limb dystonia occurs usually as an accompanying feature of cervical or axial dystonia. Isolated occurrence of non-action-induced limb dystonia is rare and usually of symptomatic origin. In children, adolescents, and young adults isolated non-action-induced limb dystonia is indicative of levodopa sensitivity and risk of spread of the symptomatology, especially when it is localised in the legs and when diurnal fluctuations are present. In non-action-induced limb dystonia pain is frequently the main complaint. Functional impairment is often of secondary importance. Especially in non-action-induced dystonia involving the leg muscles there can be a strong specific or unspecific facilitating effect of physical activity.

➤ **What are the possible target muscles in BT therapy for limb dystonia?**

The functions of the hand and finger muscles are shown in Table **20** and those of the main foot muscles in Table **21**. The possible target muscles and their recommended therapeutic BT doses are listed in Tables **22** and **23**.

Table 20 Hand muscles and finger muscles under physiological conditions

function	muscle	estimated degree of involvement
wrist extension	extensor digitorum	1
	extensor carpi radialis	2
	extensor indicis	3
	extensor pollicis longus	4
	extensor digiti minimi	5
wrist flexion	flexor digitroum superficialis	1
	flexor digitorum profundus	2
	flexor carpi ulnaris	3
	flexor pollicus longus	4
	flexor carpi radialis	5
	abductor pollicis longus	6
wrist radial abduction	extensor carpi radialis longus	1
	abductor pollicis longus	2
	extensor pollicis longus	3
	flexor carpi radialis	4
	flexor pollicis longus	5
wrist ulnar abduction	extensor carpi ulnaris	1
	flexor carpi ulnaris	2
	extensor digitorum	3
	extensor digiti minimi	4
finger extension	extensor digitorum	1
	extensor indicis	2
	extensor digiti minimi	3
finger flexion	flexor digitorum profundus	1
	flexor digitorum superficialis	1
thumb opposition	opponens pollicis	1
thumb adduction	adductor pollicis	1
thumb abduction	abductor pollicis	1

Table 21 Foot muscle functions under physiological conditions

function	muscle	estimated degree of involvement
foot extension	triceps surae	1
	peronaeus longus	2
	flexor digitorum longus	3
	flexor digitorum longus	3
	tibialis posterior	4
foot supination	triceps surae	1
	tibialis posterior	2
	flexor hallucis longus	3
	flexor digitorum longus	4
	tibialis anterior	5

Table 22 Recommended doses for botulinum toxin therapy arm muscles

muscle	function	recommended dose (100 MU-A in 2.5 ml 0.9% NaCl/H_2O) [MU-A Botox®]
deltoid	arm abduction	60 – 120
biceps brachii	forearm flexion	60 – 120
triceps brachii	forearm extension	60 – 120
bachialis	forearm flexion	60 – 120
bachioradialis	forearm flexion	60 – 100
forearm flexors	hand flexion finger flexion	30 – 100
forearm extensors	hand extension finger extension	30 – 100
interosseus	finger adduction finger abduction	20
abductor digiti quinti	little finger abduction	20 – 40
thenar muscles	thumb opposition thumb abduction thumb adduction thumb flexion	20 – 40

MU-A   mouse unit of the mouse bioassay of Allergan Inc

Table 23   Recommended doses for botulinum toxin therapy of leg muscles

muscle	function	recommended dose (100 MU-A in 2.5 ml 0.9% NaCl/H_2O) [MU-A Botox®]
adductor group	leg adduction	100 – 200
quadriceps femoris	distal leg extension	100 – 200
hamstring muscles	distal leg flexion	100 – 200
triceps surae	foot extension foot supination	80 – 160
tibialis posterior	foot supination	40 – 100
flexor hallucis longus	foot supination foot extension great toe flexion	40 – 80
tibialis anterior	foot flexion	60 – 80
extensor digitorum longus	foot flexion toe extension	40 – 60
extensor hallicus longus	foot flexion great toe extension	40 – 60

MU-A   mouse unit of the mouse bioassay of Allergan Inc

➤ **What are the difficulties of BT therapy for writer's cramp?**

BT therapy for writer's cramp is difficult because the possible target muscles have very narrow therapeutic windows. This is a problem especially in finger extensors. Additionally, writer's cramp almost always affects a large number of forearm muscles with co-contractions of all major forearm muscle groups as a common feature. BT therapy targeting all of these muscles would produce major paretic side effects and therefore should be avoided. Also, distinction between physiological and dystonic muscle activity is exceedingly difficult. This is the case since dystonic muscle activity only occurs together with physiological muscle activity, since physiological muscle activity is usually strong and often involves co-contractions similar to dystonic co-contractions, and since dystonic muscle activity frequently occurs immediately after the beginning of the physiological muscle activity. Last but not least, distinction between dystonic and compensatory muscle activity may be difficult since writer's cramp patients may compensate their dystonia with abnormal voluntary elbow and shoulder positions.

➤ **What trick can be used to distinguish between physiological and dystonic muscle activity in patients with writer's cramp ?**

In some patients with writer's cramp the dystonic muscle activity can be elicited by asking the patient to write with his non-dystonic hand. If this phenomenon is present physiological and compensatory muscle activity can easily be distinguished from dystonic muscle activity.

➤ **Which writer's cramp patients respond best to BT therapy ?**

In few patients with writer's cramp dystonia is limited to isolated muscles. These patients respond best to BT therapy, especially when electromyography is used for target muscle identification. In few other patients full dystonic muscle hyperactivity is triggered by initial hyperactivity in an isolated muscle. In these patients treatment of these trigger muscles may stop the dystonic spread and thus also yield favourable therapeutic effects without the necessity of injection into large numbers of muscles. In some cases a marked improvement of the patient's symptomatology can be achieved by administration of BT into the dystonic proximal arm and shoulder muscles which have considerably wider therapeutic windows.

➤ **What is the success rate of BT therapy for writer's cramp ?**

Because of the usually narrow therapeutic windows of the target muscles, the involvement of large numbers of forearm muscles, and difficulties in target muscle identification, the success rate of BT therapy for writer's cramp is limited. Although functional improvement is difficult to achieve, it is often possible to alleviate the patient's pain without induction of major paretic side effects. In general, optimal compromises between therapeutic effects and side effects can only be reached after several injection series. BT therapy for writer's cramp should therefore only be initiated in severe cases with marked pain after other approaches, like writing with the non-dominant hand, use of computers, and use of modified writing utensils have failed.

➤ **What is the success rate of BT therapy for action-induced limb dystonia other than writer's cramp ?**

Action-induced limb dystonias other than writer's cramp usually do not respond to BT therapy. In addition to the reasons explaining limited success rates in writer's cramp, these conditions usually occur in a functionally exceedingly complex context, thus increasing the risk of paretic side effects considerably. Rare forms of action-induced dystonia localised in leg muscles, however, bear chances of higher success rates.

Recently, the concept of using BT injections for retraining movement sequences arose amongst neurologists treating musicians with occupational cramps. As intriguing as this approach may be, it is still awaiting experimental support and clinical verification.

➤ **What is the success rate of BT therapy for non-action-induced limb dystonia ?**

In most patients with non-action-induced limb dystonia BT therapy can reduce pain substantially in both arm and leg dystonias. Improvement of functional impairment depends much on the patient's individual symptomatology. Whereas functional improvement is more difficult to achieve in arm dystonia – especially when there is associated pre-existent paresis – results in distal leg dystonia are favourable. Overall, BT therapy for non-action-induced limb dystonia is especially indicated when pain is the main complaint.

➤ **How can the effect of BT therapy for foot dystonia easily be documented ?**

The effect for BT therapy of foot dystonia can easily be documented by using a the blotting paper test. For this the patient's foot is moistened and put on a sheet of blotting paper. Several trials should be recorded. Repetition of the blotting paper test by asking the patient to just touch the blotting paper and by asking the patient to put weight on the affected foot gives information not only about the stance area but also about the mobility of the foot. Figure **28** shows the full weight stance area of a patient with foot dystonia before and after BT therapy.

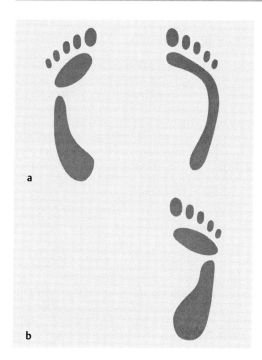

Fig. 28 Blotting paper test. Full weight stance in a patient with non-action-induced foot dystonia.
a Before botulinum toxin therapy.
b 4 weeks after botulinum toxin therapy.
From: Dressler D, Argyrakis A, Schönle PW, Wochnik G, Rüther E (1996). Botulinumtoxintherapie in der Rehabilitationsneurologie. Nervenarzt 67: 686–694.

➤ **What are the possible side-effects of BT therapy for non-action-induced limb dystonia ?**

Paretic side effects may arise especially when BT is administered in the forearm muscles because of their narrow therapeutic windows. Other muscles of the upper and lower limbs have wider therapeutic windows so that paretic side effects are less frequent. Paretic side effects are also more frequent in the presence of additional pre-existing paresis. With the high BT doses occasionally necessary for dystonia in the lower extremities the risk of systemic side effects and of BT antibody formation increases.

➤ **What other treatments are available
   when BT therapy for limb dystonia fails ?**

When BT therapy fails drug treatment may be tried, although the success rate is usually limited. Additional physiotherapy may help to prevent secondary orthopaedic complications. Sometimes positioning of the affected limb in special casts may help to prevent triggering of the dystonia. Peripheral denervation and myotomy may be helpful in some patients. Surgical central nervous system interventions should only be considered as a last option. Phenol injections can be tried in patients with BT antibody formation provided that the injector has sufficient experience with this procedure.

➤ **What additional aids may be offered
   to patients with writer's cramp ?**

At least during the early stages of the disease, some degree of improvement may be achieved by changing the motor program or the sensory feed-back of writing, by using different writing positions and by changing the grip of the writing utensil. However, the most helpful strategy is to train the use of the non-dystonic hand. About half of the patients who have learned to use the non-dystonic hand remain free of symptoms in this hand for several years. Although the other half of the patients do develop writer's cramp in the originally non-dystonic hand eventually, the onset of symptoms can be prolonged substantially in this way. Although trying to use the non-dystonic hand seems to be difficult at first, this task can usually be accomplished within a few months. The use of mechanical devices for fixating the writing utensil to the hand rather than to the fingers can be helpful in some patients.

Axial Dystonia

➤ **What is axial dystonia ?**

The term axial dystonia describes dystonic hyperactivity in muscles of the axial skeleton. These include trunk muscles and spinal muscles with the exception of neck muscles. The dystonic muscle hyperactivities lead to extensions and lateral flexions of the trunk, to torsion scoliosis and occasionally to flexions of the trunk. Axial dystonia occurs most frequently in the context of segmental or generalised dystonia. Neuroleptics-induced dystonia seems to affect axial muscles predominantly. The term "Pisa syndrome" should not be employed because of its discriminating and thus unethical nature. Isolated occurrence of an axial dystonia is rare.

➤ **What secondary damage can be caused by axial dystonia** ?

Axial dystonia induces malpositioning of the axial skeleton. This can cause discopathies with radicular lesions as well as arthrosis of vertebral joints. After prolonged and severe courses, deformations of the thoracic and abdominal cavities can occur and may give rise recurrent pneumonia and cardiac arrhythmias.

➤ **What are the possible target muscles in BT therapy for axial dystonia** ?

The possible target muscles and their recommended BT doses are listed in Table **24.** In most cases BT is administered to the spinal muscles but occasionally muscles of the abdominal wall may also serve as target muscles. Since large muscle groups are often affected in axial dystonia and since the total BT dose that can be used is limited, it is important to focus the BT therapy on the most affected sites and to ensure that these sites receive sufficient BT doses.

Table 24 Recommended doses for botulinum toxin therapy of axial muscles

muscle	function	recommended dose (100 MU-A in 2.5 ml 0.9% NaCl/H_2O) [MU-A Botox®]
paravertebral muscles (1 segment)	sagittal trunk extension ipsilateral frontal trunk flexion	60 – 80 per side

MU-A   mouse unit of the mouse bioassay of Allergan Inc

➤ **What is the success rate of BT therapy for axial dystonia** ?

Because of the generally wide-spread dystonic involvement and the limited total BT dose that may be used, residual dystonic symptoms can usually still be detected after BT therapy for axial dystonia. However, with careful target muscle selection and use of appropriate BT doses in these target muscles, BT therapy usually results in marked improvement of the condition.

➤ **What are the possible side effects
of BT therapy for axial dystonia** ?

Paretic side effects of BT therapy for axial dystonia are extremely rare, since paravertebral muscles have a broad therapeutic window. Since high BT doses are usually required in BT therapy for axial dystonia systemic side effects may occur in isolated cases. These side effects only last for a few days and do not constitute major impairment for the patient.

➤ **What other treatments are available
when BT therapy for axial dystonia fails** ?

As in other forms of dystonia the first alternative is drug treatment. In addition, physiotherapy may help to alleviate the patient's symptomatology. Central nervous system surgery should only be considered as a last resort. Epidural spinal electrostimulations are of uncertain efficacy. Continuous intrathecal baclofen administration may prove to be helpful in those patients.

Generalised Dystonia

➤ **What is generalised dystonia** ?

The term generalised dystonia describes dystonic hyperactivity affecting at least three extremities and the axial muscles. Generalised dystonia usually starts focally and then spreads during the further course of the condition. In adults, generalisation of focal dystonia is very rare. In children, adolescents, and young adults, however, there is a considerable risk of generalisation. This juvenile onset generalised dystonia is clinically distinct from generalised dystonia first occurring in adults. In juvenile onset dystonia many patients exhibit typical diurnal fluctuations of their symptomatology. Administration of levodopa can improve this condition dramatically. In most forms of generalised dystonia the symptomatology consists of pain and functional impairment of the affected muscles. This impairment can become dramatic especially in long-lasting conditions. In the final stage patients are bed-ridden and unable to sit up or to use any of their extremities. Food intake can be limited by violent cervical and pharyngeal dystonia. Respiration may be impaired by scoliotic changes of the thorax caused by axial dystonia as well as by dystonic spasms of the respiratory muscles, by pharyngolaryngeal dystonia, and by cervical dystonia. In the final stage the patient's life is endangered by repeated attacks of pneumonia and cardiac arrhythmias.

➤ **What is the role of BT therapy
in the treatment of generalised dystonia ?**

BT therapy is not the therapy of choice for generalised dystonia. Emphasis should first be placed on drug treatment. When there is sufficient evidence of diurnal fluctuations, levodopa should be given. In patients with focal, juvenile onset, generalised dystonia without typical diurnal fluctuations the success rate of levodopa treatment is low, but given the benign character of this drug a trial should be performed. For conclusive testing the levodopa dose should be in the order of 600 mg/d given over a period of at least 3 months. Only when drug therapy fails, which unfortunately is very often the case, should BT therapy be initiated. Except for occasionally successful stereotactic procedures, surgical interventions have not shown any significant effect and thus should be taken into consideration, if at all, only after a BT therapy. Continuous intrathecal baclofen application is a new approach currently being investigated.

➤ **What are the difficulties with
BT therapy for generalised dystonia ?**

The major problem with BT therapy for generalised dystonia results from the large number of affected muscles. Since the total BT dose that can be given is limited successful treatment depends on careful target muscle selection.

➤ **What are the possible target muscles
in BT therapy for generalised dystonia ?**

In principle, all muscles that can be used as target muscles in BT therapy for focal dystonia may also be used as possible target muscles in BT therapy for generalised dystonia. Since generalised dystonia is affecting numerous muscles and since the total BT dose that can be given is limited it is of paramount importance to focus BT therapy in this condition. Target muscle selection depends on the focus of the patient's impairment. Suitable target muscles are usually those muscles causing pain. Target muscle selection can also be helped by input from physiotherapy or nursing.

➤ **What is the success rate of BT therapy for generalised dystonia ?**

Because of the large number of muscles affected and the limited BT dose applicable the success rate of BT therapy for generalised dystonia is limited. However, careful target muscle selection and administration of sufficiently high BT doses into these target muscles can lead to considerable improvements. This applies especially to pain.

➤ **What are the possible side effects**
  of BT therapy for generalised dystonia ?

In principle, possible side effects of BT therapy for generalised dystonia do not differ from possible side effects of BT therapies for corresponding focal dystonia. Since higher BT doses are used in BT therapy for generalised dystonia, mild systemic side effects such as shortness of breath, fits of perspiration, a general feeling of fatigue, accommodation deficiencies, dry mouth, and dysphagias may sometimes occur. In general, these side effects last for few days only. However, the use of excessively high total BT doses is strongly contraindicated. BT therapy for generalised dystonia should be carried out by specially experienced physicians only. The first treatment should be performed as an in-patient procedure.

➤ **What other treatments are available**
  if BT therapy for generalised dystonia fails ?

If BT therapy for generalised dystonia fails, drug treatment and physiotherapeutic interventions can alleviate the patient's symptomatology. For severe forms, stereotactic procedures may be helpful. Epidural spinal electrostimulation is of limited efficacy. Continuous intrathecal baclofen application is a new approach currently being investigated.

Spastic Conditions

➤ **What are spastic conditions** ?

We have suggested the term spastic conditions to clarify terminological uncertainties arising from the notoriously undifferentiated use of the term spasticity in clinical practice. The term spastic conditions describes different forms of muscle stiffness occurring together with paresis after acute lesions of the central nervous system as frequently seen in rehabilitation neurology. Table **25** summarises the different spastic conditions.

spasticity
spasm
rigidity
dystonia
alpha rigidity
gegenhalten
guarding
contracture

Table 25   Spastic conditions

➤ **What is spasticity** ?

The term spasticity describes involuntary muscle hyperactivity of short duration which occurs exclusively on rapid passive stretching of the respective muscle.

➤ **What is rigidity** ?

The term rigidity describes involuntary muscle hyperactivity which occurs on slow passive stretching of the respective muscle.

➤ **What is spasm** ?

The term spasm describes endogenously- or exogenously-induced prolonged involuntary muscle hyperactivity.

➤ **What is alpha rigidity?**

The term alpha rigidity describes continuous muscle hyperactivity at rest producing a typical "plastic" rigidity.

➤ **What is gegenhalten?**

The term gegenhalten describes involuntary muscle activity maintaining positions of body parts against exogenous force.

➤ **What is guarding?**

The term guarding describes voluntary muscle activity maintaining positions of body parts to avoid pain.

➤ **What is contracture?**

The term contracture describes limitations of passive joint mobility. They can be caused by shortening of tendons, shrinkage of joint capsules and muscle alterations. Contractures are not associated with muscle hyperactivity.

➤ **What are the differential diagnoses of spastic conditions?**

Apart from spastic conditions, muscle stiffness can be due to a number of conditions. Most of them are very rare. Muscle stiffness can be caused by peripheral nervous system dysfunctions, such as myokymia, neuromyotonia, pseudomyotonia, Isaac syndrome and Schwartz-Jampel syndrome. These conditions are not accompanied by paresis nor are they due to lesions of the central nervous system. Muscle stiffness can also be caused by muscular dysfunctions, such as myopathies, myotonias and water and electrolyte imbalances. Again, none of these conditions is due to lesions of the central nervous system. Muscle stiffness can be caused by dysfunctions of GABAergic spinal interneurons as in stiff person syndrome, or other spinal interneurons as in tetanus and strychnine poisoning. However, paretic features do not occur in these conditions. Muscle stiffness may also be caused by various forms of cerebral or spinal inflammation including progressive encephalomyelitis with rigidity or spinal interneuronitis, encephalitis lethargica, *Borrelia burgdorferi* infection, by neoplasms including paraneoplastic syndromes, and by infarction and haemorrhage. Whether these conditions cause spastic conditions with acute muscle stiffness and paresis or isolated muscle stiffness depends on their localisation. Muscle stiffness due to spontaneous or hereditary degenerative or metabolic processes both have a non-acute course.

Abnormal posturing of body parts can be caused by postural apraxia and by focal polymyositis resembling dystonia but lacking of any muscle hyperactivity.

➤ **What central nervous system structures are damaged in spastic conditions** ?

Spastic conditions are produced by combined lesions of pyramidal and extrapyramidal structures within the central nervous system. Extrapyramidal lesions can be intracerebral affecting the basal ganglia and their input and output pathways or intraspinal affecting descending pathways. Intraspinal interneurons do not seem to be affected in spastic conditions.

➤ **What pathological processes can cause spastic conditions** ?

Spastic conditions can be caused by various pathological processes of the central nervous system, most frequently by infarctions, haemorrhages, trauma and inflammations including encephalomyelitis disseminata. Tumour as a cause is less common.

➤ **How can spastic conditions be documented** ?

Spastic conditions can be documented with respect to spastic and rigid muscle tone, to spasm frequency, muscle power and global care impairment induced as shown in Tables **26** to **30** (Appendix, p. 140 – 141).

➤ **Which spastic conditions respond to BT therapy** ?

BT therapy can be successfully applied for dystonia and rigidity. Spasms can also be alleviated to a certain extent by BT therapy. Pain in these cases responds especially well to BT therapy. Functional deficiencies can also improve under BT therapy. First experience suggests that contractures may possibly respond partially to BT therapy, although it is not clear what mechanisms would be involved.

➤ **Which spastic conditions do not respond to BT therapy** ?

Although BT therapy can reduce muscle hyperactivity in spasticity, this does not have a major impact on the clinical symptomatology because the duration of the spastic muscular hyperactivity is all together very short and the muscle hyperactivity practically never produces pain. Gegenhalten also does not respond to BT therapy because its muscular hyperactivity is not limited to specific target muscles. Postural apraxia sometimes mimicking spastic conditions cannot be treated by BT therapy since it is associated with muscle hypoactivity rather than with muscle hyperactivity.

➤ **How should the BT therapy for spastic conditions be planned** ?

Exact analysis of patient's complaint is the key step in planning BT therapy for spastic conditions. Physiotherapists, nursing staff, and family members should also report their observations and list their ideas about possible therapy objectives. After a particularly thorough neurological examination, the treatment objectives have to be defined. They should balance therapeutic wishes and limitations of BT therapy due to dose limitations and obligatory local side effects. BT therapy for spastic conditions is more than in any other indication highly individualised to the clinical symptomatology and the individual situation of the patient. It requires a substantial degree of experience.

➤ **What are typical treatment objectives**
  of BT therapy for spastic conditions ?

BT therapy for spastic conditions can be useful to treat pain, to improve functional deficits and cosmetic deficits, to facilitate physiotherapeutic exercise programmes, further rehabilitation strategies, and nursing care.

➤ **What treatment objectives can be achieved best** ?

Of all treatment objectives, reduction of pain can be achieved best. In most cases almost complete elimination of pain should be possible. Functional, cosmetic, physiotherapeutic, and nursing care improvement can usually only be partially achieved. However, this can mean a substantial improvement of the patient's condition.

➤ **What are the possible target muscles for BT therapy for spastic conditions ?**

All limb muscles may be used as target muscles in BT therapy for spastic conditions. The individual target muscle selection depends on the treatment objectives defined for the individual patient.

➤ **What are the possible side effects of BT therapy for spastic conditions ?**

In principle, the possible side effects of BT therapy for spastic conditions are the same as those for other BT therapy indications in respective muscles. In contrast to other indications for BT therapy, however, by definition pareses of the target muscles pre-exists in spastic conditions. Obviously, this increases the risk of paretic side effects from BT therapy. The risk of systemic side effects is also higher because BT therapy for spastic conditions generally involves higher BT doses than BT therapy for other conditions.

➤ **When is BT therapy for spastic conditions particularly successful ?**

BT therapy for spastic conditions is particularly successful when the voluntary strength of the target muscles is only slightly decreased, so that the obligatory BT-induced weakening of the target muscles is functionally not significant. BT therapy for spastic conditions is also particularly successful when the voluntary strength of the target muscle is decreased to an extent that additional BT-induced weakening does not further reduce the patient's functional abilities.

➤ **When is BT therapy for spastic conditions less successful ?**

BT therapy for spastic conditions is less successful when the voluntary power of the target muscles is already reduced to an intermediate extent so that any additional weakening of the target muscles produces additional functional deficits.

➤ **What are the conventional treatment options for spastic conditions ?**

Spastic conditions can be treated conventionally with oral drugs, such as benzodiazepam, tizanidine, baclofen, or dantrolene, or with continuous intrathecal administration of baclofen. Orthopaedic surgery and phenol neurolysis can also be helpful. Avoidance of noxious stimuli and physiotherapy should be applied to all patients. Serial casting can be tried to regain passive mobility, whereas positional casting may help to avoid trigger positions of the limbs.

Cerebral Palsy

➤ **What is cerebral palsy ?**

The term cerebral palsy, or Little's disease, describes a wide spectrum of pyramidal dysfunctions, extrapyramidal dysfunctions, and apraxic disorders that are caused by perinatal brain damage. The pyramidal dysfunctions manifest as central paresis, while extrapyramidal dysfunctions produce spasticity, rigidity, dystonia, spasms, and chorea. Reduced growth of affected limbs, contractures, and joint lesions are frequently observed. They often produce pain, which can become the leading symptom. The term cerebral poliomyelitis, sometimes used as a synonym for cerebral palsy, is misleading since it suggests a non-existent relationship to poliomyelitis. Although cerebral palsy is caused by acute perinatal damage, it may change over time because of complex interactions between the static lesion and multiple dynamic growth and compensation processes.

➤ **What is the experience with BT therapy for cerebral palsy ?**

BT therapy for cerebral palsy has many features in common with BT therapy for spastic conditions. Looking at the single elements of extrapyramidal dysfunction in cerebral palsy, the use of BT therapy for cerebral palsy becomes apparent. For the single elements of extrapyramidal dysfunction, the same therapeutic principles as for their isolated occurrence in adults apply. Obviously, BT doses have to be adjusted to the lower body weight of children. So far, BT doses used in children correspond closely to the body weight-corrected BT doses used in adults.

BT therapy for cerebral palsy is mainly used to produce functional improvement. For this, hyperactivities of calf muscles and adductor muscles are treated. Muscle hyperactivities in the upper extremity have been treated occasionally. In most of the patients with leg disability, clinically important gait improvements can be achieved. BT administration into arm muscles is less successful and it may be accompanied by paretic side effects. Evidence available so far suggests that early initiation of BT therapy for cerebral palsy can prevent the development of contractures and other secondary lesions. It can normalise further growth of the affected limb. Pyramidal dysfunction is not improved by BT treatment. BT treatment may, in fact, produce paretic side effects.

Apart from functional improvement, BT therapy for cerebral palsy can be very successfully used for the treatment of pain caused by muscle hyperactivity. This can be very helpful for the management of pain after release surgery. BT may also be used to plan orthopaedic surgery in cerebral palsy by providing a tool for temporary testing the effect of these procedures.

BT therapy for cerebral palsy can be combined with conventional treatment of cerebral palsy. Where and how different treatment strategies are complementing each other, has not been evaluated yet.

Tremor

➤ What is tremor?

The term tremor describes involuntary muscle hyperactivity occurring at regular intervals in time.

➤ What is the role of BT therapy in the management of tremor?

BT therapy for tremor is not the treatment of choice for this condition and should only be considered after all possible drug treatments have been tried.

➤ Which forms of tremor can be managed by BT therapy?

Since BT therapy for tremor is a purely symptomatic treatment, all forms of tremor can, in principle, be treated by BT therapy.

➤ Which forms of tremor are difficult to treat with BT therapy?

As with BT therapy for dystonia, treatment of tremor with BT is difficult when the muscle hyperactivity causing tremor is localised in multiple muscles and when it is localised in muscles with narrow therapeutic windows. Treatment of limb tremors, therefore, is on the whole rather disappointing.

➤ Which forms of tremor respond best to BT therapy?

Tremor responds best to BT when the muscle hyperactivity causing tremor is localised in few muscles and when it is localised in muscles with a wide therapeutic window. Head tremor, jaw tremor, and palatal tremor, therefore respond favourably to BT therapy.

➤ What is the success rate of BT therapy for tremor?

In head tremor substantial improvements of the symptomatology can be achieved in many patients. Especially secondary phenomena, such as vertigo, impaired fixation, and feelings of tension respond well, whereas the extent of head excursions itself may still be noticeable. Success rates and the side effects of BT therapy for jaw tremor are similar to those of BT therapy for bruxism. BT therapy for palatal tremor requires considerably manual experience and is often accompanied by side effects.

➤ What are the possible side effects of BT therapy for tremor?

BT therapy for head tremor and jaw tremor can be accompanied by the same side effects as BT therapy for the corresponding dystonias. BT therapy for palatal tremor can produce severe dysphagia and speech impairment.

Hemifacial Spasm

➤ **What is hemifacial spasm ?**

The term hemifacial spasm describes involuntary hyperacitivity of mimic muscles. At the onset of the condition this muscle hyperactivity typically consists of short muscle twitches. Later on, the muscle twitches occur in series and confluence to tonic muscle spasms. Usually symptoms are noticed first in the periocular muscles. Later on they involve cheek muscles and muscles of the corner of the mouth. When the muscle twitches occur in more than one mimic muscle, their occurrence is always synchronous. Hemifacial spasm is practically always limited to only one side of the face. Bilateral hemifacial spasm exists but is extremely rare. If it does occur the muscle twitches are not synchronous in both sides of the face.

➤ **What is the aetiology of hemifacial spasm ?**

Hemifacial spasm arises from a dysfunction of the peripheral nervous system. Hemifacial spasm is not a form of dystonia. Based on intraoperative findings it is assumed that hemifacial spasm results from an irritation of the facial nerve caused by small aberrant vessels adjacent to the facial nerve immediately after its exit from the brain stem. Pulsations of the blood flow in these vessels cause chronic irritation of the facial nerve tissue with ephaptic discharges. In the further course of the condition about one third of the patients suffer from discrete paresis manifesting predominantly in the muscles of the corner of the mouth.

➤ **What is the conventional treatment of hemifacial spasm ?**

Hemifacial spasm can conventionally be treated by drugs or by neurosurgical interventions.

➤ **What is the drug treatment of hemifacial spasm ?**

Drug treatment of hemifacial spasm with carbamazepine or phenytoin attempts to stabilise axonal membranes. For both drugs the same serum levels as for anticonvulsive indications are aimed at. About one third of the patients treated in this way will respond with a reduction of their symptomatology. However, this improvement is only partial and transient. Occasionally, side effects such as a tiredness or slowed reactions can occur. Restrictions regarding the use of motor vehicles have to be observed.

➤ **What is the neurosurgical therapy for hemifacial spasm ?**

The neurosurgical treatment of hemifacial spasm is the neurolysis operation according to *Jannetta*. In this procedure, a retroauricular approach is used to expose the exit region of the facial nerve. Under microscopic control a tissue pad is then placed between the facial nerve and a vessel loop found there in all patients operated on so far. The success rate of the *Jannetta* operation is impressive. Practically every patient responds with an almost complete remission and this remission does not appear to be limited in duration. Re-occurrences of the symptoms can happen when the tissue pad is dislocated. Side effects of the *Jannetta* operation are rare, but when they occur, they can be serious. Sensory and motor hemisyndromes as well as acoustic and vestibular impairments have been reported. Despite the impressive results and the low frequency of side-effects, patients only rarely decide to undergo this operation because of the relative mild nature of their disorder.

➤ **What are the possible target muscles
in BT therapy for hemifacial spasm ?**

Figure **17** (p. 54) shows the mimic muscles. The possible target muscles and their recommended therapeutic BT doses are listed in Table **9** (p. 55). For treatment of hemifacial spasm BT is usually administered into the periocular muscles as for blepharospasm. Administration of BT in the perioral muscles is less frequently used. In this case muscles of the chin and lower lip area, such as the mentalis and the depressor labii inferioris, are particularly suitable. Muscles in the cheek, such as the risorius muscle, may also be used, but careful adjustment of BT dosages is necessary to avoid dysfunction of the corner of the mouth.

➤ **What are the difficulties of BT therapy
in target muscles of the lower face ?**

As with BT therapy for Meige syndrome, the narrow therapeutic windows of muscles in the lower face have to be remembered. Thus, injection of BT into these target muscles can easily produce functionally disturbing paretic side effects. BT dosing in these muscles must therefore be made with extreme caution. Paretic side effects, especially with perioral injections, occur more frequently than those after BT therapy for

Meige syndrome because of underlying clinical or subclinical facial pareses frequently arising after chronic irritation of the facial nerve.

➤ **Which muscles should be avoided in BT therapy for hemifacial spasm**?

As with BT therapy for Meige syndrome, all muscle elevating the corner of the mouth, such as the levator labii superiores, the levator angulis oris, and the zygomatic muscles, should not be used as target muscles. Also, injections of BT into the orbicularis oris muscle in the upper lip should be avoided.

➤ **What is the success rate of BT therapy for hemifacial spasm**?

In almost all patients treated the periocular muscular hyperactivity can be abolished resulting in normalisation of vision and reduction of muscular tension. In the cheek and mouth regions muscular hyperactivity is frequently reduced, even when BT is given strictly periocularly. The reason for this phenomenon is not clear. It is assumed to be due to local diffusion processes. Speculations that periocular muscles could act as trigger muscles for muscles in the cheek and mouth regions have not been confirmed experimentally so far. Figure **29** shows a typical treatment profile of a patient with hemifacial spasm.

➤ **What is the duration of BT therapy for hemifacial spasm**?

The effect of BT therapy for hemifacial spasm lasts on average for about four to five months. Thus, this duration is about one month longer than that of blepharospasm. So far, this phenomenon has not been explained. It can be speculated that the underlying paresis of mimic muscles, often seen in hemifacial spasm, may either cause relative overdosing or that it may slow down the re-innervation process.

➤ **What are the possible side-effects of BT therapy for hemifacial spasm**?

Periocular administration of BT for hemifacial spasm can, in principle, produce the same side effects as BT therapy for blepharospasm. The perioral administration of BT can, despite the above-mentioned precautionary measures, lead to paresis of the corner of the mouth, paraesthesias, and lip instabilities.

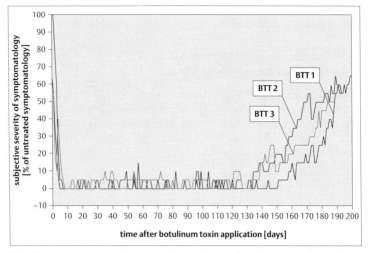

Fig. 29   Treatment profile of a patient with hemifacial spasm and botulinum toxin therapy. The profile was reconstructed based on the treatment calendar shown in Fig. **9** (Appendix, p. 128).

BTT 1   botulinum toxin therapy, first application
BTT 2   botulinum toxin therapy, second application
BTT 3   botulinum toxin therapy, third application

➤ **What is the role of BT therapy
   in the management of hemifacial spasm ?**

BT therapy for hemifacial spasm has one of the highest success rates and one of the lowest frequencies of side effects of all conditions treated with BT. Usually, patients started on BT therapy do not wish to try drug treatment or to undergo the *Jannetta* operation. It may be discussed whether progression of paresis of the corner of the mouth and young age might be reasons to undergo surgery rather than use BT therapy.

Facial Synkinesias

> **What are facial synkinesias** ?

The term synkinesia describes involuntary muscular activities caused by peripheral nerve damage with misdirected sprouting and therefore faulty re-innervation. Although synkinesias can, in principle, arise in any part of the body, only facial synkinesias are of clinical relevance. Despite the relatively high frequency of facial nerve dysfunction, facial synkinesias are a rare phenomenon. Their clinical features are involuntary co-activation of muscles of the corner of the mouth when activation of the eyelid closure muscles is intended and vice versa. These co-activations do not constitute a serious functional problem, but they can be cosmetically disturbing and often lead to feelings of muscular tension.

Although few in total number, synkinesias are an obligate side effect of hypoglossofacial anastomosis operations, which become occasionally necessary when the facial nerve was lesioned in cerebellopontine angle operations. In these patients, involuntary co-activation of many of the facial muscles occurs when activation of lingual muscles is intended for mastication or swallowing. Although synkinesias after hypoglossofacial anastomoses can initially lead to substantial functional and cosmetic problems, central compensatory mechanisms may lead to gradual remission of the initial symptomatology.

> **What are the possible target muscles
> in BT therapy for facial synkinesias** ?

Figure **17** (p. 54) shows the mimic muscles. The possible target muscles and their recommended therapeutic BT doses are listed in Table **9** (p. 55). Most frequently, periocular muscles are chosen, whereas perioral muscles are less frequently used. In synkinesias after hypoglossofacial anastomosis, both periocular and perioral muscles may be target muscles for BT therapy.

> **What are the limitations of target muscle
> selection in BT therapy for facial synkinesias** ?

In BT therapy for facial synkinesias the same limitation apply as in BT therapy for hemifacial spasm.

➤ **What are the specific difficulties
of BT therapy for facial synkinesias ?**

BT therapy for facial synkinesias is complicated by obligate residual paresis due to the primary disease process. To avoid paretic side effects, BT doses, therefore, have to be considerably lower than the BT doses used for treatment of blepharospasm.

➤ **What is the success rate of BT therapy for facial synkinesias ?**

The success rate of BT therapy for facial synkinesias is lower than the success rate of BT therapy for blepharospasm because of the frequent involvement of perioral muscles. Apart from the genuinely narrow therapeutic window of these muscles, further restrictions arise from obligate residual pareses due to the primary disease process. In general, most patients experience some degree of reduction of their complaints, of which the feelings of tension seem to respond best.

Facial Asymmetries

➤ **How can facial asymmetries be caused ?**

Facial asymmetries can be caused by facial paresis due to facial nerve lesions and central pareses. In particular, pathological processes in the cerebellopontine angle can produce persistent and severe facial nerve lesions causing cosmetically and functionally very disturbing asymmetry between the paretic and the non-paretic side of the face.

➤ **What are the possible target muscles
in BT therapy for facial asymmetries ?**

Figure **17** (p. 54) shows the mimic muscles. The possible target muscles in BT therapy for facial asymmetries are the mimic muscles of the non-paretic side of the face. These possible target muscles and their recommended BT doses are listed in Table **9** (p. 55). BT therapy for this indication is intended to produce partial paresis of the non-paretic side of the face resembling the original contralateral residual paresis.

➤ **What is the success rate of BT therapy for facial asymmetries?**

BT therapy for facial asymmetries can balance the primarily non-paretic and the primarily paretic side of the face with consecutive improvement of cosmetic appearance and overall functioning.

➤ **What are the possible side effects of BT therapy for facial asymmetries?**

The possible side effects of BT therapy for facial asymmetries correspond to those of BT therapy for Meige syndrome.

Strabismus

➤ **What is strabismus?**

The term strabismus describes a misalignment of the optical axes of the eyeballs with impairment of binocular vision.

➤ **What are the causes of strabismus?**

Strabismus can be caused by disorders of central gaze control as in concomitant strabismus where central fusion mechanisms are impaired, either permanently or in certain gaze positions only. Very often patients with concomitant strabismus have absent or poor binocular function, either acutely or due to compensation mechanisms occurring years after the acute event. Lesions of one or several peripheral nerves, frequently caused by head trauma in road traffic accidents, can produce paralytic strabismus. Restrictive strabismus is caused by space-occupying processes within the orbita, whereas muscular strabismus occurs in myopathy and myositis of external eye muscles.

➤ **What are the possible target muscles in BT therapy for strabismus?**

The possible target muscles for BT therapy for strabismus are the straight external eye muscles. Oblique external eye muscles have not been injected so far.

➤ **How is BT therapy for strabismus performed ?**

BT administration is performed with a combined EMG injection cannula, which is inserted into the belly of the target muscle. For horizontal straight external eye muscles access is gained through the conjunctiva, which is prepared by local anaesthetics and vasoconstrictors. BT injections into vertical straight external eye muscles are performed transcutaneously. Local anaesthetics and vasoconstrictors are not needed for this procedure. Exact positioning of the injection cannula is controlled by simultaneously recording the EMG signal of the target muscle. The combined EMG-injection cannula is shown in Figure **27** (p. 79). In children intravenous ketamine anaesthesia may be used.

➤ **What are the indications in BT therapy for strabismus ?**

BT therapy for strabismus can be used to treat concomitant strabismus, paralytic strabismus, restrictive strabismus, and muscular strabismus. It can also be used for predict the outcome of strabismus surgery as well as to optimise its outcome.

➤ **What is the principle of BT therapy for strabismus ?**

The principle of BT therapy for strabismus is to compensate eyeball malpositions by producing paresis of external eye muscles. Since prolonged paresis of the external eye muscles can produce permanent contractures in the antagonistic muscles, it was hoped that BT therapy for strabismus could achieve the same effect, thus inducing permanent improvement of the condition treated. When BT therapy for strabismus was actually tried, contractures of the antagonistic muscles could hardly be induced. However, in patients with mild or moderate squints, fusion stabilised permanently after several BT injection series. Therefore, in contrast to other indications, BT therapy for strabismus is planned as a temporary intervention to re-set fusion.

In BT therapy for paralytic strabismus, BT is given into the antagonists of the paretic muscles to lengthen them for prevention of contractures.

> ➤ **What is the experience with BT therapy for concomitant strabismus ?**

Since almost all patients with concomitant strabismus have absent or poor binocular function, BT therapy for concomitant strabismus is aimed at a cosmetic improvement rather than a functional improvement. For minor eyeball deviations several series of BT therapy may permanently improve the squint by inducing slight contractures in muscles antagonistic to the target muscles. For more pronounced eyeball deviations improvement of the squint will only be temporary and surgery is therefore preferable. Frequently, BT therapy is used as a adjunct to strabismus surgery when overcorrection or undercorrection occurs. When the postoperative squint is small or moderate the chances are high that several series of BT therapy may produce a permanent correction. For larger squints, the chances for a permanent improvement are lower.

BT administration can also be used to test whether cosmetic surgery for concomitant strabismus will produce postoperative diplopia. It seems that BT therapy is more helpful for this purpose than conventional optical tests. When concomitant strabismus is caused by temporary interruption of vision in one eye, BT administration can help to determine whether surgery can restore binocular function.

> ➤ **What is the experience with BT therapy for paralytic strabismus ?**

Of all forms of strabismus, paralytic strabismus is probably the best indication for the use of BT therapy. In paralytic strabismus, BT is mainly used for prevention of contractures in antagonist muscles of the paretic muscles. Although definite studies on the ultimate outcome of paralytic strabismus are still lacking, BT therapy shortens the duration of strabismus and decreases its severity. BT therapy for prevention of contractures, obviously, should be initiated without much delay after the acute event. Several series of BT therapy can also improve chronic paralytic strabismus. For this purpose, squints have to be relatively mild and fusion has to be intact. It seems that acute paralytic strabismus responds better than chronic forms.

In paretic strabismus, BT administration can help to distinguish between residual partial paresis and contracture of its antagonist muscle. For this purpose, the development of a short acting BT preparation would be helpful. BT administration together with transposition surgery can improve the outcome of the procedure, especially with respect to ischaemic complications.

➤ **What is the experience with BT therapy for restrictive strabismus ?**

The therapy of choice for restrictive strabismus is treatment of the underlying cause. However, restrictive strabismus can be treated successfully with BT administrations in cases in which causal treatment cannot be performed or has to be delayed.

➤ **What is the experience with BT therapy for muscular strabismus ?**

BT therapy can be used successfully to compensate muscular strabismus due to thyroid disease. This is particularly helpful when strabismus surgery cannot be performed due to active thyroid dysfunction. Strabismus resulting from extraocular eye muscle scarring and sensory deprivation after retinal detachment surgery or cataract surgery can be improved by BT treatment. BT therapy has not yet been reported in patients with myopathic strabismus.

➤ **What are the possible side effects of BT therapy for strabismus ?**

As with strabismus surgery, overcompensations and undercompensations of the squint angle can arise after BT therapy for strabismus. In rare cases, transient ptosis can occur. Intraorbital haemorrhage and bulbus perforation cannot be excluded completely, but are very rare events.

Protective Ptosis

➤ **What is protective ptosis?**

The term protective ptosis describes an intentional iatrogenic eyelid closure for therapeutic reasons. Protective ptosis is used in the therapy for ulcerating keratitis which would not heal in the absence of eyelid closure.

➤ **How can protective ptosis be induced conventionally?**

Protective ptosis is conventionally induced by tarsorhaphy in which the eyelids are sutured together.

➤ **What are the possible side effects of tarsorhaphy?**

Tarsorhaphy can induce permanent damage to the eyelid margins, sometimes severely interfering with lacrimation dynamics.

➤ **What are the possible target muscles in BT administration for protective ptosis?**

The target muscle for BT administration for protective ptosis is the levator palpebrae muscle.

➤ **What is the success rate for BT administration for protective ptosis?**

Complete eyelid closure for a period of about three months can easily be produced by BT administration. Unlike with tarsorhaphy BT induced protective ptosis allows direct access to the cornea at any time. The duration of BT-induced protective ptosis usually corresponds favourably with the duration of eyelid closure required for healing.

➤ **What are the possible side effects of BT-induced protective ptosis?**

Side effects of BT induced protective ptosis have not been observed so far. Normal functioning of the levator palpebrae will be regained since BT does not produce permanent alterations in its target muscles.

Entropion

➤ **What is entropion?**

The term entropion describes the inversion of the margins of the eyelid towards the eyeball with consecutive irritation of the cornea and the conjunctiva by the eyelashes. It is caused by loosening of the connective tissue of the eyelids with displacement of the orbicularis oculi muscle to the margin of the eyelid with consecutive inversion of the eyelid. Since this process is almost exclusively seen with ageing, entropion is often referred to as senile entropion. Entropion caused by hyperactivity of the orbicularis oculi muscle in blepharospasm and acute eye irritations is called spastic entropion. Among our patients with blepharospasm spastic entropion is a rare condition.

➤ **What are the possible target muscles
   in BT therapy for entropion?**

The target muscle in BT therapy for entropion is the orbicularis oculi muscle. Since entropion normally occurs in the lower eyelid, BT is usually given into the portion of the orbicularis oculi muscle in the lower eyelid.

➤ **What is the success rate of BT therapy for entropion?**

BT therapy for entropion can almost always achieve improvement. However, the degree of improvement is variable, with patients with spastic entropion responding better than those with senile entropion. The therapeutic effect usually lasts for about three months.

➤ **What are the possible side-effects of BT therapy for entropion?**

The possible side effects of BT therapy for entropion are similar to those of BT therapy for blepharospasm with the exception that ptosis is not to be expected since BT injections are restricted to the lower eyelid. Paretic ectropion does not seem to appear with the usual therapeutic dosages.

➤ **What is the role of BT therapy in the management of entropion?**

The role of BT therapy in the management of entropion has not been clarified, since long-term experience is not yet available and comparative studies with surgical treatment, which is effective and permits definitive treatment, have not yet been performed.

➤ **Can BT therapy be used for the management of ectropion ?**

BT therapy is contraindicated in cases of senile ectropion since this condition is caused by a loosening of the connective tissue of the eyelid or by paresis of the orbicularis oculi muscle. In both cases BT administration into the orbicularis oculi muscle would worsen the condition.

Exocrine Gland Hyperactivity

➤ **What exocrine gland hyperactivities have been treated with BT so far ?**

So far, BT has been used for Frey syndrome, crocodile tears syndrome, and for focal forms of hyperhidrosis.

➤ **Why is the BT application for exocrine gland hyperactivity constituting a novel aspect of BT use ?**

BT application for exocrine gland hyperactivity constitutes a novel aspect of BT use because it represents the first use of BT in non-muscular target tissues. In all three exocrine gland hyperactivity syndromes, BT blocks the muscarinic acetylcholine synapses of the parasympathetic or sympathetic autonomic nerve fibres stimulating exocrine gland secretion.

➤ **How can exocrine gland hyperactivity be documented ?**

Focal hyperactivity of sweat glands can for most purposes be localised by clinical observation. For this the suspected skin area is dried thoroughly. When the sweat production starts the produced sweat will change the light reflection of the hyperhidrotic area so that it can be localised easily. For photographic demonstration and planimetric evaluation the starch iodine test according to Minor can be used. This test is described in Table **31**. Practical problems with this test include accidental spreading of sweating borders by the application of Lugol's solution and wash out effects due to overexposure or due to profuse sweating. The ninhydrine test can be used to document palmar and plantar hyperhidrosis. Gravimetric tests are measuring the weight of the produced

Table 31   Starch iodine test according to Minor

cleaning and drying of skin

application of Lugol's solution (J_2 3.0, KJ 6.0, H_2O ad 150.0) with swap stick

application of starch with dispenser

waiting until blue-coloration of starch is maximal

sweat soaked into a piece of paper tissue. With all tests control of environmental and body temperatures, humidity, air flow, preceding physical activity and emotional state are crucial but difficult to guarantee.

➤ **What is Frey syndrome ?**

The term Frey syndrome describes excessive sweating, sometimes associated with flush and paraesthesias, which usually affects the temporal areas of the skull. Often it is localised in the skin areas innervated by the auriculotemporalis nerve or the auricularis magnus nerve. Frey syndrome occurs six to twelve months after parotid gland operations when parasympathetic fibres of the facial nerve originally innervating the parotid gland are re-sprouting into the adjacent skin and its sweat glands. A similar process has been observed after resections of the submandibular gland. When saliva production is stimulated by specific taste or smell sensations, such as sour taste or other intense sensations, these aberrant nerve fibres stimulate excessive sweating rather than salivation. Because of the linkage between taste sensations and the induction of sweating this phenomenon is also known as gustatory sweating. Although Frey syndrome is harmless, it can be cosmetically disturbing.

➤ **What is the conventional treatment of Frey syndrome ?**

Conventional treatment options include systemic application of anticholinergics, skin excision, chemical or surgical dissections of the auriculotemporalis and auricularis magnus nerves, radiation of the skin, obstruction of the sweat gland ducts with aluminium chloride (aluminium chloride 15.0, methyl cellulose 2.0, aqua demineralisata ad 100.0, to be applied onto the affected skin every second night), and application of local anaesthetics to the oral mucosa. Probably the most successful strategy is to prophylactically isolate the skin with a fascia lata interponate when parotid operations are performed.

➤ **How is BT application for Frey syndrome performed** ?

BT application for Frey syndrome is performed by intracutaneous injection of BT into the affected skin where it blocks the muscarinic acetylcholine synapses of the sympathetic innervation of the sweat glands. Usually 4 mouse units of Botox® (Botox® 100 mouse units diluted with 5.0 ml 0.9% NaCl/H_2O) injected into one site of an area of 4 cm^2 should produce sufficient blockade of hyperhidrosis. Higher doses may be used if necessary. Skin areas covering sensitive mimic muscles should be avoided to prevent paretic side effects.

➤ **What is the experience with BT application for Frey syndrome** ?

BT application should normalise hyperhidrosis in Frey syndrome in all patients treated. So far therapy failure for this indication has not been reported. Occasionally tissue penetration of the BT applied is not sufficient so that islands of hyperhidrotic skin persist. Then additional injections should be performed. With the dosis used for Frey syndrome stimulation of BT antibody formation is not to be expected. The duration of the therapeutic effect for this indication sometimes exceeds 12 months. Exsiccotic skin irritation does not occur.

➤ **What is crocodile tears syndrome** ?

The term crocodile tears syndrome describes eccessive unilateral lacrimation during eating. To spoil crocodile's tears originates from the assumption that crocodiles are weeping whilst swallowing their prey thus pretending false compassion. It was first used as a medical term by the Russian neurologist Bogorad from Minsk in 1928. Crocodile tears syndrome occurs after proximal facial nerve lesions when re-sprouting of parasympathetic nerve fibres originally inducing salivation is misdirected into the lacrimal glands. When saliva production is stimulated lacrimation is then induced. Crocodile tears syndrome is harmless, but can be cosmetically disturbing.

➤ **What is the conventional treatment of crocodile tears syndrome** ?

Conventional treatment consists of resection of the lacrimal gland with consecutive risk of keratoconjunctivitis sicca and of temporary or permanent blockade of the ganglion sphenopalatinum, which is technically difficult and sometimes yields temporary or partial relief only.

➤ **How is BT application for crocodile tears syndrome performed ?**

BT application for crocodile tears syndrome is performed by injection of BT directly into the upper part of the lacrimal gland where it blocks the muscarinic acetylcholine synapses of its sympathetic innervation. By asking the patient to adduct the eye and by spreading the eye lids apart the target area can easily be located in the external angle of the eye. Usually 4 mouse units of Botox® (Botox® 100 mouse units diluted with 5.0 ml 0.9% NaCl/H$_2$O) injected into one site should produce sufficient blockade of excessive lacrimation.

➤ **What is the experience with BT application for crocodile tears syndrome ?**

BT application should normalise excessive lacrimation in crocodile tears syndrome in all patients treated. So far therapy failure for this indication has not been reported. The duration of the therapeutic effect for this indication is about 6 months. Keratoconjunctivitis sicca does not occur. Other side effects, such as diplopia and ptosis, seem to be rare. BT antibody formation is not to be expected.

➤ **What is hyperhidrosis ?**

The term hyperhidrosis describes excessive sweating. Hyperhidrosis is estimated to affect approximately 1% of the general population. It can occur generalised or focal. Generalised hyperhidrosis is in most cases of idiopathic origin. Often there is a positive family history. Occasionally it can be caused by anxiety disorders, infections, malignancies, endocrinologic disorders, drugs and by hypothalamic lesions. Focal hyperhidrosis is also usually of idiopathic origin with genetic factors. Symptomatic forms can be due to anxiety disorders and to irritations of central or peripheral autonomic pathways. Despite some anatomical insight most of the physiology and pathophysiology of sweating is not yet understood.

➤ **What is the conventional treatment of hyperhidrosis ?**

Conventional treatment of hyperhidrosis includes systemic application of anticholinergics, local application of aluminium chloride (aluminium chloride 15.0, methyl cellulose 2.0, aqua demineralisata ad 100.0, to be applied onto the affected skin every second night) for obstruction of the sweat gland ducts, local application of tannine and iontophoresis. Peripheral, transthoracic or endoscopic sympathetic blockades and dissections, axillar skin excisions and axillar subcutaneous curettages have also been tried. In the relatively few cases of symptomatic hyperhidrosis correction of the underlying condition is indicated. Additionally, application of beta blockers, appropriate clothing with a high natural fibre content and avoidance of intensive spices and of alcohol may be helpful. Generally, non-surgical methods are effective only to a limited degree whilst surgical procedures bear the risk of side effects.

➤ **How is BT application for hyperhidrosis performed ?**

BT application for hyperhidrosis is performed by intracutaneous injection of BT into the affected skin where it blocks the muscarinic acetylcholine synapses of the sympathetic innervation of the sweat glands. Usually 4 mouse units of Botox® (Botox® 100 mouse units diluted with 5.0 ml 0.9% NaCl/H_2O) injected into one site of an area of 4 cm^2 produces sufficient blockade of hyperhidrosis. Higher doses may be used if necessary. The number of injection sites vary from 10 to 15 in axillar hyperhidrosis to 15 to 25 in palmar hyperhidrosis. Experience with BT application for platar hyperhidrosis is still anecdotal. In generalised hyperhidrosis only few affected skin areas can be targeted. Since the palmar and for some reason even more so the plantar skin are rather pain sensitive tissues BT application into these skin areas is somewhat unpleasant. For palmar BT application local anaesthetic blocks of the median and ulnar nerves have been suggested, but from our experience their benefit does not outweigh their disadvantages. Local anaesthetic cremes are not producing sufficient benefit since they are only affecting pain fibres on the surface of the skin but not in its deeper structures. BT application into the plantar skin are sometimes unpleasant enough to prevent patients from pursuing this treatment. To avoid BT wash out from the highly perfused target tissue we apply a pressure cuff inflated with pressures well above the systolic blood pressure. This procedure, together with a straight forward performance of the procedure, reduces discomfort to an acceptable level.

➤ **What is the experience with BT application for hyperhidrosis ?**

BT application for axillar hyperhidrosis is regularly producing complete blockade of hyperhidrosis. Side effects are not to be expected. Treatment of palmar hyperhidrosis is more difficult since the total hyperhidrotic skin area is increased by interdigital involvement and some transient hand weakness can occur. It also seems that the diffusion properties of the palmar skin and especially the plantar skin are less favourable than the diffusion properties of the axillar skin. The duration of the therapeutic effect is in the order of 3 to 4 months. BT antibody formation has not been reported so far, but may be possible depending on the doses used.

➤ Can BT applications be used for relative hypersalivation ?

Relative hypersalivation occurs when the substantial amounts of saliva continuously produced throughout the day cannot be swallowed properly. This may be the case in motor neuron disease, Parkinson's disease and in bulbar and pseudobulbar paresis. When BT is injected into the parotid glands relative hypersalivation is stopped without induction of dryness of mouth. BT doses necessary are in the order of 40 mouse units of Botox® (Botox® 100 mouse units diluted with 5.0 ml 0.9 % NaCl/H_2O). Additional injections of the sublingual and submandibular glands are rarely necessary.

➤ Can BT applications be used for rhinorhea ?

Animal experiments and preliminary applications in patients indicate that BT might be used in the future for therapy of refractory rhinorhea.

Detrusor Sphincter Dyssynergia

➤ What is detrusor sphincter dyssynergia ?

The term detrusor sphincter dyssynergia describes an impaired interaction of the urinary bladder muscles with relative hyperactivity of the urethral sphincter muscle, usually caused by lesions of the spinal cord. It leads to incomplete bladder voiding with recurrent urinary tract infections and secondary urinary incontinence. Drug therapies, urinary condoms, intermittent or permanent catheterisation, electrostimulation, and sphincterotomies have been suggested for its management. Satisfactory treatment results, however, are difficult to obtain.

➤ **What is the target muscle of BT administration for detrusor sphincter dyssynergia?**

The target muscle of BT administration for detrusor sphincter dyssynergia is the striated sphincter urethrae muscle. An anatomically definable sphincter of the bladder wall itself does not exist. The sphincter urethrae muscle can be accessed either transcutaneously through the perineum or transurethrally. In both cases identification of the target muscle and injection of BT is performed with an EMG cannula.

➤ **What is the experience with BT administration for detrusor sphincter dyssynergia?**

In most cases BT administration for detrusor sphincter dyssynergia results in a pronounced reduction of urinary retention. As with sphincterotomies, adequate function of the detrusor vesicae muscle is a prerequisite for satisfactory treatment results.

➤ **Can BT administrations be used for isolated bladder sphincter spasms?**

BT administration can be used for isolated bladder sphincter spasms in the same way as for detrusor sphincter dyssynergia.

Anismus

➤ **What is anismus?**

The term anismus describes a recurrent constipation possibly induced by dystonic muscle hyperactivity of the anal sphincter. Conventional treatment with high doses of laxatives, myectomies of the anal sphincters, and subtotal colotomies is effective only in a small number of patients.

➤ **What is the experience with BT administration for anismus?**

First trials of BT injection into the puborectal muscle have shown substantial improvement of anismus. Therapy results obtained with BT administration appear to be superior to those obtained with surgery especially since incontinence could be avoided.

Anal Fissures

➤ **What is the experience with BT administration for chronic anal fissures ?**

Patients with chronic anal fissures are suffering from a vicious circle: pain due to infection of anal fissures induces spasms of the external anal sphincter which in turn prevent healing of the fissures. Conventional therapy for chronic anal fissures, therefore, consists of surgical splitting of the external anal sphincter with all its accompanying side effects. First results suggest that temporary relaxation of the external anal sphincter by BT injections can break this vicious circle and initiate healing. With this approach persistent morphological changes to this sensitive organ can be avoided. Incontinence does not seem to be a major side effect. As with other indications for BT therapy, if it does occur at all, it is temporary.

Vaginismus

➤ **What is the experience with BT administration for vaginismus ?**

The term vaginismus describes involuntary hyperactivity of vaginal and perianal muscles preventing penile penetration during intercourse. Although the precise aetiology of this condition is unknown, behavioural therapy or progressive dilator therapy usually helps. In therapy refractory cases, however, BT injection into the anterior vaginal wall may help for periods of several months.

Achalasia

➤ **What is achalasia ?**

The term achalasia describes a hyperactivity of the lower oesophageal sphincter. Although a dysfunction of inhibitory neurons of the myenteric plexus (Auerbach's plexus) in the oesophageal wall is assumed, the exact cause of this condition is not yet known.

➤ **What is the target muscle in BT administration for achalasia ?**

When BT is used to manage achalasia it is injected directly into the anatomical correlate of the lower oesophageal sphincter.

➤ **What is the experience with BT administration for achalasia ?**

So far there are only few reports on the use of BT for achalasia. However, these reports indicate that a reduction of the hyperactivity of the lower oesophageal sphincter can be achieved without induction of major side effects. The effectivity of BT for this indication can be elegantly demonstrated by measurements of the intraoesophageal pressure.

➤ **Why does the administration of BT
for achalasia constitute a novel aspect of BT use ?**

BT administration for achalasia constitutes a novel aspect of BT use because it represents the first use of smooth muscles as target tissue for BT therapy. BT apparently blocks the muscarinic acetylcholine synapses of the parasympathetic vagus nerve.

Hyperactive Facial Lines

➤ **What is the experience with BT administration
for hyperactive facial lines ?**

The term hyperactive facial lines is used to describe wrinkles caused by muscle hyperactivity of mimic muscles. Classically, they occur as craw's feet around the lateral epicanthus and as frowning in the forehead. Despite fierce polypragmatic and notoriously expensive attempts by cosmetic surgeons and the cosmetic industry to abolish them, virtually nothing is known about their aetiology. Success rates of conventional interventions are poor and their possible side effects are sometimes horrifying. After individual patients have reported positive effects of BT on their hyperactive facial lines after they received BT for blepharospasm or hemifacial spasm, the use of BT for this purpose is becoming increasingly fashionable amongst certain cosmetic surgeons and their clients. To be amenable for BT administration the wrinkles have to be caused by muscle hyperactivity. If that is the case BT administration for wrinkles should be successful in the periorbital and frontal area.

For BT administration for perioral wrinkles the same limitations as for BT therapy for perioral dystonia apply.

If wrinkles are caused by connective tissue alterations they will not respond or get worse after BT administration. If wrinkles are caused by muscle hyperactivity and if this muscle hyperactivity has caused connective tissue alterations the cosmetic effect might be unfavourable. Even if the cosmetic effect of BT administration in itself is favourable, the changed facial expression will be unusual to people surrounding the client and some time will be necessary for them to get familiar to the altered facial expression.

Nystagmus

➤ **What is the experience with BT administration for nystagmus?**

BT injections into the lateral rectus muscles can suppress nystagmus. However, severe double vision often arises as a side effect. For this reason BT therapy for nystagmus is only indicated for severe cases. Additional eye coverage for suppression of double vision can be tried.

Gilles de la Tourette Syndrome

➤ **What is the experience with BT administration for Gilles de la Tourette syndrome?**

The term Gilles de la Tourette syndrome describes the combination of brief involuntary movements and short explosive and often obscene vocalisations. Associated features include obsessive-compulsive behaviour. BT administration into the vocal cords in Gilles de la Tourette syndrome has been tried in a few patients with malignant, socially devastating vocalisations to induce aphonia. Surprisingly, in those patients treated the urge to produce vocalisations was reduced without induction of aphonia. The mechanism for this is unknown. BT injections have also been tried with promising results in patients with dystonic, i.e., prolonged, cervical ticks. It seems that the more tonic the muscle hyperactivity is the better the outcome may be.

Tardive Dyskinesia

➤ **What is the experience with BT administration for tardive dyskinesia ?**

The term tardive dyskinesia describes the broad spectrum of movement disorders seen during or after treatment with neuroleptic drugs. BT administration has been successful when dystonic elements are identified. Choreartic, athetoid, or tremor elements hardly respond to BT. Obviously the particular aetiology of the muscle hyperactivity treated with BT does not seem to matter.

Postoperative Immobilisation

➤ **What is the experience with BT administration for postoperative immobilisation ?**

BT administration can be used after operations to immobilise muscles, joints, tendons and their insertions for ensuring improved healing. For this purpose, BT has only been used in individual patients with dystonia in the operation field in which an operation would not have been possible without BT immobilisation. Whether BT immobilisation can be helpful for operations in patients without dystonia needs to be assessed.

Appendix

Fig. 9   Treatment calendar for patients with movement disorders based upon the patient's self assessment. ▶

Treatment Calendar for Patients with Movement Disorders

patient name

type of movement disorder

How to use this calendar...

1. This calendar helps to monitor the severity of your movement disorder over the time. This is very important information for your physician to plan your therapy properly. Therefore your cooperation is in your own interest.

2. Please, fill out this calendar every evening before you go to bed.

3. To fill out this calendar, please, circle the percent-value that best describes the severity of your movement disorder symptomatology for that particular day.

4. 0% describes the condition where you do not have any movement disorder symptomatology at all. 100% describes the condition you experienced before any therapy was started for the first time. 100% would also describe the condition when botulinum toxin therapy would not work at all. For all other conditions, please, circle the percent-figure you believe is appropriate.

5. Quite understandably, it must seem to you rather difficult to abstractly describe your movement disorder symptomatology to a precision of as much as 5%. However, with some practice this precision allows you to record very subtle changes of your symptomatology on a day to day basis.

6. In the column remarks you can note everything you consider remarkable.

7. Please, bring this calendar to every physician's appointment.

Month:

Movement Disorder Symptomatology
(in percent of maximal untreated symptomatology)

Day																						Remarks
1	0	5	10	15	20	25	30	35	40	45	50	55	60	65	70	75	80	85	90	95	100	
2	0	5	10	15	20	25	30	35	40	45	50	55	60	65	70	75	80	85	90	95	100	
3	0	5	10	15	20	25	30	35	40	45	50	55	60	65	70	75	80	85	90	95	100	
4	0	5	10	15	20	25	30	35	40	45	50	55	60	65	70	75	80	85	90	95	100	
5	0	5	10	15	20	25	30	35	40	45	50	55	60	65	70	75	80	85	90	95	100	
6	0	5	10	15	20	25	30	35	40	45	50	55	60	65	70	75	80	85	90	95	100	
7	0	5	10	15	20	25	30	35	40	45	50	55	60	65	70	75	80	85	90	95	100	
8	0	5	10	15	20	25	30	35	40	45	50	55	60	65	70	75	80	85	90	95	100	
9	0	5	10	15	20	25	30	35	40	45	50	55	60	65	70	75	80	85	90	95	100	
10	0	5	10	15	20	25	30	35	40	45	50	55	60	65	70	75	80	85	90	95	100	
11	0	5	10	15	20	25	30	35	40	45	50	55	60	65	70	75	80	85	90	95	100	
12	0	5	10	15	20	25	30	35	40	45	50	55	60	65	70	75	80	85	90	95	100	
13	0	5	10	15	20	25	30	35	40	45	50	55	60	65	70	75	80	85	90	95	100	
14	0	5	10	15	20	25	30	35	40	45	50	55	60	65	70	75	80	85	90	95	100	
15	0	5	10	15	20	25	30	35	40	45	50	55	60	65	70	75	80	85	90	95	100	
16	0	5	10	15	20	25	30	35	40	45	50	55	60	65	70	75	80	85	90	95	100	
17	0	5	10	15	20	25	30	35	40	45	50	55	60	65	70	75	80	85	90	95	100	
18	0	5	10	15	20	25	30	35	40	45	50	55	60	65	70	75	80	85	90	95	100	
19	0	5	10	15	20	25	30	35	40	45	50	55	60	65	70	75	80	85	90	95	100	
20	0	5	10	15	20	25	30	35	40	45	50	55	60	65	70	75	80	85	90	95	100	
21	0	5	10	15	20	25	30	35	40	45	50	55	60	65	70	75	80	85	90	95	100	
22	0	5	10	15	20	25	30	35	40	45	50	55	60	65	70	75	80	85	90	95	100	
23	0	5	10	15	20	25	30	35	40	45	50	55	60	65	70	75	80	85	90	95	100	
24	0	5	10	15	20	25	30	35	40	45	50	55	60	65	70	75	80	85	90	95	100	
25	0	5	10	15	20	25	30	35	40	45	50	55	60	65	70	75	80	85	90	95	100	
26	0	5	10	15	20	25	30	35	40	45	50	55	60	65	70	75	80	85	90	95	100	
27	0	5	10	15	20	25	30	35	40	45	50	55	60	65	70	75	80	85	90	95	100	
28	0	5	10	15	20	25	30	35	40	45	50	55	60	65	70	75	80	85	90	95	100	
29	0	5	10	15	20	25	30	35	40	45	50	55	60	65	70	75	80	85	90	95	100	
30	0	5	10	15	20	25	30	35	40	45	50	55	60	65	70	75	80	85	90	95	100	
31	0	5	10	15	20	25	30	35	40	45	50	55	60	65	70	75	80	85	90	95	100	

Table 6 Standardised video protocol for documentation of dystonia in various body parts

region	recording position	conditions	approximate recording time [s]
head	from front	looking straight at camera at normal light	60
		looking straight at camera and counting backwards	45
		looking straight at camera with forced repetitive fist closures	30
		10 forced voluntary repetitive eye closures with consecutive looking straight into bright light	30
		reading small print	30
neck	from front	spontaneous head position during unsupported sitting	60
		5 smooth voluntary maximal head rotations to right and left	30
		spontaneous head position during unsupported sitting with counting backwards	45
		spontaneous head position during unsupported sitting with repetitive fist closures	30
		spontaneous head position during walking on the spot	30
		forced walking over 30 m	90
	from right side, left side, back	spontaneous head position during unsupported sitting	60
		5 smooth voluntary maximal head rotations to right and left	30
trunk	from front	spontaneous trunk position during unsupported sitting	60
		forced walking over 30 m	60
	from front, one side and back	spontaneous trunk position during walking on the spot	90

Table 6 Standardised video protocol for documentation of dystonia in various body parts *(continuation)*

region	recording position	conditions	approximate recording time [s]
arms	from front	resting arms in lap	60
		holding arms in front of chest with fingers of both hands pointing towards each other	
		tapping all fingers consecutively on thumb	30
		writing standard sentence in normal handwriting	30
		writing standard sentence in print	45
		copying objects	45
		drawing spiral from inward to outward with arm resting on elbow	30
		10 forced repetitive fist closures with consecutive spreading fingers apart	30
legs	from front	spontaneous sitting	60
		walking on the spot	30
		forced walking over 30 m	60

Table 7 Dystonic movement rating scale for generalised dystonia. Focal dystonia can be rated when the weight factor is abandoned; modified from: Burke RE, Fahn S, Marsden CD, Bressman SB, Moskowitz C, Friedman J (1985) Validity and reliability of a rating scale for the primary torsion dystonias. Neurology 35: 73 – 77

region	provoking factor (A)	severity factor (B)	weight factor (C)	score
eyes	0 no dystonia at rest or with action 1 dystonia on particular action 2 dystonia on many actions 3 dystonia on action of distant body parts or intermittently at rest 4 dystonia present at rest	0 no dystonia present 1 occasional blinking 2 frequent blinking without prolonged eye closure 3 prolonged eye closure, but eyes open most of the time 4 prolonged eye closure with eyes closed at least 30 % of the time	0.5	([A + B] × C)
mouth	0 no dystonia at rest or with action 1 dystonia on particular action 2 dystonia on many actions 3 dystonia on action of distant body parts or intermittently at rest 4 dystonia present at rest	0 no dystonia present 1 occasional grimacing or other mouth movements 2 dystonia present less than 50 % of the time 3 moderate dystonia present most of the time 4 severe dystonia present most of the time	0.5	([A + B] × C)
speech swallowing	0 normal 1 occasional dystonia 2 frequent dystonia either on speech or on swallowing 3 frequent dystonia on speech or swallowing together with occasional dystonia on speech or swallowing 4 frequent dystonia on speech and swallowing	0 normal 1 speech easily understood or occasional choking 2 speech occasionally difficult to understand or frequent choking 3 speech understandable with difficulties only or inability of swallowing solid foods 4 complete anarthria or marked difficulty swallowing soft foods or liquids	1.0	([A + B] × C)
neck	0 no dystonia at rest or with action 1 dystonia on particular action 2 dystonia on many actions 3 dystonia on action of distant body parts or intermittently at rest 4 dystonia present at rest	0 no dystonia present 1 occasional pulling 2 mild but obvious torticollis 3 moderate pulling 4 extreme pulling	0.5	([A + B] × C)

Table 7 Dystonic movement rating scale for generalised dystonia   (continuation)

region	provoking factor (A)	severity factor (B)	(C)	score
right arm	0 no dystonia at rest or with action 1 dystonia on particular action 2 dystonia on many actions 3 dystonia on action of distant body parts or intermittently at rest 4 dystonia present at rest	0 no dystonia 1 slight and clinically insignificant dystonia 2 obvious but not disabling dystonia 3 ability to grasp preserved 4 no useful grasp	1.0	([A + B] × C)
left arm	0 no dystonia at rest or with action 1 dystonia on particular action 2 dystonia on many actions 3 dystonia on action of distant body parts or intermittently at rest 4 dystonia present at rest	0 no dystonia 1 slight and clinically insignificant dystonia 2 obvious but not disabling dystonia 3 ability to grasp preserved 4 no useful grasp	1.0	([A + B] × C)
trunk	0 no dystonia at rest or with action 1 dystonia on particular action 2 dystonia on many actions 3 dystonia on action of distant body parts or intermittently at rest 4 dystonia present at rest	0 no dystonia 1 slight and clinically insignificant bending 2 definite bending not interfering with standing and walking 3 moderate bending interfering with standing and walking 4 extreme bending preventing from standing and walking	1.0	([A + B] × C)
right leg	0 no dystonia at rest or with action 1 dystonia on particular action 2 dystonia on many actions 3 dystonia on action of distant body parts or intermittently at rest 4 dystonia present at rest	0 no dystonia 1 clinically not significant dystonia 2 dystonia with brisk and unaided walking 3 dystonia with severely impaired walking 4 dystonia with inability to walk and to stand	1.0	([A + B] × C)
left leg	0 no dystonia at rest or with action 1 dystonia on particular action 2 dystonia on many actions 3 dystonia on action of distant body parts or intermittently at rest 4 dystonia present at rest	0 no dystonia 1 clinically not significant dystonia 2 dystonia with brisk and unaided walking 3 dystonia with severely impaired walking 4 dystonia with inability to walk and to stand	1.0	([A + B] × C)

Table 8 Dystonia disability rating scale for generalised dystonia. Focal dystonia can be rated when the weight factor is abandoned; modified from: Burke RE, Fahn S, Marsden CD, Bressman SB, Moskowitz C, Friedman J (1985) Validity and reliability of a rating scale for the primary torsion dystonias. Neurology 35: 73 – 77

function	quantification (A)	weight factor (B)	score
pain	0 not occurring 1 mild, less 2 hours/day 2 mild, more than 2 hours/day 3 severe, less 2 hours/day 4 severe, more than 2 hours/day	5	(A × B)
stance	0 not impaired 1 impaired, but possible without external support 2 impaired, but possible only with mechanical devices 3 impaired, but possible only with supporting person 4 not possible	4	(A × B)
locomotion	0 not impaired 1 impaired, but possible without external support 2 impaired, but possible with mechanical devices 3 impaired, but possible with supporting person 4 not possible	4	(A × B)
speech	0 not impaired 1 impaired, but easily understood 2 some difficulty in understanding 3 marked difficulty in understanding 4 complete or almost complete anarthria	4	(A × B)

Table 8 Dystonia disability rating scale (*continuation*)

function	quantification (A)	weight factor (B)	score
eating	0 not impaired 1 impaired, but possible 2 impaired, but possible with choking 3 impaired, but possible with supporting person 4 impaired, but possible with supporting person and with choking	4	(A × B)
sleep	0 not impaired 1 impaired falling asleep 2 waking up at night	3	(A × B)
secondary alterations	0 not detectable 1 haematoma 2 nerve entrapment syndromes 2 skin laceration 3 orthopaedic alterations 3 reactive depression 5 suicidal thoughts 5 cardiac arrhythmias 5 pulmonary complications	3	(A × B)
writing	0 not impaired 1 impaired, but legible 2 almost legible 3 illegible 4 inability to grasp or maintain hold on pen	2	(A × B)

Table 8 Dystonia disability rating scale for generalised dystonia *(continuation)*

function	quantification (A)	weight factor (B)	score
hygiene	0 not impaired 1 self hygiene with effort 2 hygiene with external support 3 hygiene with external support substantial effort necessary 4 adequate hygiene not possible	2	(A × B)
dressing	0 not impaired 1 clumsy, but independent 2 help necessary for some activities 3 help necessary for most activities	1	(A × B)

Table 16   Standard passage for testing of spasmodic dysphonia

The north wind and the sun

The north wind and the sun were arguing one day about which of them was the stronger, when a traveller came along, wrapped in a warm coat. They agreed that the one who could make the traveller take off his coat would be considered stronger than the other one. Then the north wind blew as hard as he could, but the harder he blew the tighter the traveller wrapped his coat around him. And at last the north wind gave up trying. Then the sun began to shine warmly, and right away the traveller took off his coat. And so the north wind had to admit that the sun was stronger than he was.

Table 17   Assessment protocol for spasmodic dysphonia according to Whurr et al. (Whurr R, Lorch M, Fontana H, Brookes G, Lees A, Marsden CD (1993) The use of botulinum toxin in the treatment of adductor spasmodic dysphonia. J Neurol Neurosurg Psychiat 56: 526–530)

1	read standard passage (see Table **16**) with normal volume
2	cough
3	breath in
4	breath out (sigh)
5	whisper count from one to five
6	hum "Mmmmm"
7	say "Ah" in a low pitch
8	say "Ah" in a high pitch
9	glide up on a scale on "La"
10	glide down on a scale on "La"
11	pitch "Ah" low then high
12	pitch "Ah" high then low
13	count from one to ten in alternating pitch
14	shout "Taxi"
15	read standard passage (see Table **16**) with loud volume
16	conversation

Table 18 Unified spasmodic dysphonia rating scale (USDRS) after Stewart et al. (Stewart CF, Allen EL, Tureen P, Diamond BE, Blitzer A, Brin MF (1997) Adductor spasmodic dysphonia: standard evaluation of symptoms and severity. J Voice 11: 95 – 103)
a Conversational speech and rating form

description	score
overall severity	1 2 3 4 5 6 7
rough voice quality	1 2 3 4 5 6 7
breathy voice quality	1 2 3 4 5 6 7
strained-strangled voice quality	1 2 3 4 5 6 7
abrupt voice initiation	1 2 3 4 5 6 7
voice arrest	1 2 3 4 5 6 7
aphonia	1 2 3 4 5 6 7
voice loudness	1 2 3 4 5 6 7
bursts of loudness	1 2 3 4 5 6 7
voice tremor	1 2 3 4 5 6 7
expiratory effort	1 2 3 4 5 6 7
speech rate	1 2 3 4 5 6 7
speech intelligibility reduced	1 2 3 4 5 6 7
related movements and grimaces	1 2 3 4 5 6 7
(circle all that apply, then rate the most severe one and mark it with an asterisk)	
	total score

scale

1 no instance
2 mild
3 mild-to-moderate
4 moderate
5 moderate-to-severe
6 severe
7 profound

definitions

overall severity is an estimate of the global severity of the voice and speech disorder
rough voice quality is an abnormal voice quality that sounds harsh, hoarse, raspy, coarse, or uneven
breathy voice quality is an abnormal voice quality with audible escape of turbulent air and weak phonation
strained-strangled voice quality is an abnormal voice quality that is squeezed and effortful
abrupt voice initiation is an abnormal initiation of phonation where sound is produced by first stiffening the vocal folds then adducting the vocal folds to the midline, building up pressure below the glottis, and finally initiating phonation; an explosive sound called the glottal attack

Table 18 Unified spasmodic dysphonia rating scale (USDRS) *(continuation)*

definitions *(continuation)*

voice arrest is an abnormal unexpected interruption in voice production during a voiced sound, suggesting either the impedance of airflow by the vocal cords closing too tightly, or the reverse, a decrease in resistance to airflow by a sudden opening of the vocal folds

aphonia is an abnormal involuntary whisper or loss of voice

abnormal voice loudness is the volume or intensity of a sound; an involuntary abnormality observed when the voice is insufficiently or excessively loud

bursts of loudness are an abnormal involuntary sudden increase or decrease in loudness

voice tremor is an abnormal involuntary voice quality of rapidly occurring fluctuations in pitch and/or loudness resulting in a quavering sound similar to a vibrato

expiratory effort is an impression of involuntary increased resistance to the flow of air during speech; an involuntary in crease in perceived labour in the production of phonation

speech rate is the speed of producing utterances; reduced speed is related to lengthened consonants and vowels or to unexpected pauses between sounds, syllables, or words; increased speed is related to shortened consonants and vowels or decreased pauses between phrases and sentences

speech intelligibility reduced is the quality of overall clarity with which an utterance can be understood or comprehended by the average listener

related movements and grimaces are the involuntary visible changes in a patient's body that accompany effortful speech including flushing of the face, facial tics such as lip movements, eye-blinking, and frowning; and movements in the neck, shoulder, arm, and leg

b Voice and speech task rating form

task	within normal limits	not within normal limits	comments
say a sustained "Ah"			
say a sustained "E"			
make your voice go up and down			
say a sustained "E" in falsetto			
whisper "Shh, the baby is sleeping"			
loudly say "Taxi"			

Table 26   Spasticity score according to Ashworth (Ashworth B [1964] Preliminary trial of carisoprodol in multiple sclerosis. Practitioner 192: 540–542)

score	description
1	no increase in muscle tone
2	slight increase in muscle tone, giving a "catch" when affected part is moved in flexion or extension
3	more marked increase in muscle tone but affected limb easily flexed
4	considerable increase in muscle tone, passive movement difficult
5	affected limb rigid in flexion or extension

Table 27   Spasm frequency score according to Penn (Penn RD [1988] Intrathecal baclofen for severe spasticity. NY Acad Sci 531: 157–166)

score	description
0	no spasms
1	mild spasms induced by stimulation
2	infrequent full spasms occurring less than once per hour
3	spasms occurring more than once per hour
4	spasms occurring more than 10 times per hour

Table 28   Rigidity rating scale from the Unified Parkinson's Disease Rating Scale (Fahn S, Elton RL [1987] Members of the UPDRS Development Committee. In: Koller WC [ed] Handbook of Parkinson's Disease. Dekker, New York)

score	description
0	absent
1	slight or detectable only when activated by mirror or other movements
2	mild to moderate
3	marked, but full range of motion easily achieved
4	severe, range of motion achieved with difficulty

Judgment on passive movement of major joints with patient relaxed in sitting position ignoring cogwheeling.

Table 29 Muscle power rating scale according to the Medical Research Council (Medical Research Council [1976] Aids to the examination of the peripheral nervous system. Memorandum 45. HMSO, London)

score	description
0	no visible contraction
1	visible contraction only
2	contraction moves joint but not against gravity
3	contraction moves joint against gravity but not against resistance
4	contraction moves joint against resistance
5	normal

Table 30 Global care impairment scale according to Dressler et al. (Dressler D, Argyrakis A, Schönle PW, Wochnik G, Rüther E [1996] Botulinumtoxinthe-rapie in der Rehabiltationsneurologie. Nervenarzt 67: 686 – 694)

score	description
1	care not impaired
2	self care with effort
3	care with one assistant
4	care with one assistant with effort
5	care with two assistants
6	care with two assistants with effort
7	no adequate care possible

Bibliography

During the last years the literature on BT therapy has grown dramatically as illustrated in Figure **30** and originates from a wide variety of countries as shown in Figure **31**.

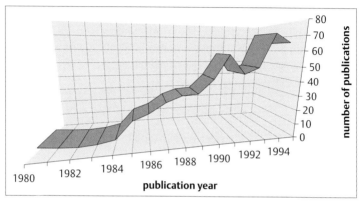

Fig. 30 Number of publications on the therapeutic use of botulinum toxin according to Medline™.

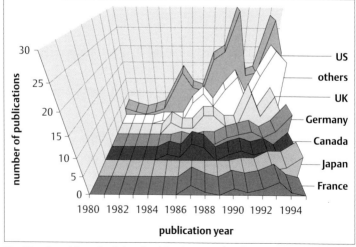

Fig. 31 Countries of origin of publications on the therapeutic use of botulinum toxin according to Medline™

This bibliography is intended to serve as a database to find references for the most common topics of BT therapy. It is a selection of references published up to December 1999. Under each topic, the references are listed according to their publication year and within each year alphabetically according to the first author's names. A reference may appear under more than one headline if it is relevant to more than one topic.

Titles given in square brackets are English translations of the originals.

I **Basic Principles of Botulinum Toxin Therapy**

1 **Mode of Action**

1.1 **Morphological Studies**

The action of botulinum toxin at the neuromuscular junction. Sellin LC. Med Biol. 1981; 59: 11–20

Pathological changes in levator palpebrae superioris muscle treated with botulinum toxin in a case of carotico-cavernous fistula. Adams GG, Dilly PN. Br J Ophthalmol. 1991; 75: 181–4

Innervation zone of orbicularis oculi muscle and implications for botulinum A toxin therapy. Borodic GE et al. Ophthal Plast Reconstr Surg. 1991, 7: 54–60

Ultrastructural changes in the masseter muscle of Macaca fascicularis resulting from intramuscular injections of botulinum toxin type A. Capra NF et al. Arch Oral Biol. 1991; 36: 827–36

Histologic features of human orbicularis oculi treated with botulinum A toxin. Harris CP et al. Arch Ophthalmol. 1991; 109: 393–5

Proton magnetic resonance spectroscopic studies of hypertrophied muscle. Effect of botulinum toxin treatment. Narayana PA et al. Invest Radiol. 1991; 26: 58–64

Effects of repeated botulinum toxin injections on orbicularis oculi muscle. Borodic GE, Ferrante R. J Clin Neuroophthalmol. 1992; 12: 121–7

Histologic assessment of dose-related diffusion and muscle fiber response after therapeutic botulinum A toxin injections. Borodic GE et al. Mov Disord. 1994; 9: 31–9

Botulinum toxin A prevents the development of contractures in the hereditary spastic mouse. Cosgrove AP, Graham HK. Dev Med Child Neurol. 1994; 36: 379–85

Botulinum toxin treatment in the facial muscles of humans: evidence of an action in untreated near muscles by peripheral local diffusion. Eleopra R et al. Neurology 1996; 46: 1158–60

Effects of botulinum neurotoxin type A on abducens motoneurons in the cat: ultrastructural and synaptic alterations. Pastor AM et al. Neuroscience 1997; 81: 457–78

1.2   Neurophysiological Studies

Botulinum toxin for blepharospasm: single-fiber EMG studies. Sanders DB et al. Neurology 1986; 36: 545 – 7

The effects of botulinum toxin on hemifacial spasm: an electrophysiologic investigation. Laskawi R et al. Ear Nose Throat J. 1990; 69: 704 – 5, 709 – 11, 715 – 7

Eyelid movements before and after botulinum therapy in patients with lid spasm. Manning KA et al. Ann Neurol. 1990; 28: 653 – 60

Botulinum-induced alteration of nerve-muscle interactions in the human orbicularis oculi following treatment for blepharospasm. Alderson K et al. Neurology 1991; 41: 1800 – 5

Quantitative electromyographic analysis of changes in muscle activity following botulinum toxin therapy for cervical dystonia. Buchman AS et al. Clin-Neuropharmacol. 1993; 16: 205 – 10

Electromyographic single motor unit potentials after repeated botulinum toxin treatments in cervical dystonia. Odergren T et al. Electroencephalogr Clin Neurophysiol. 1994; 93: 325 – 9

Quantitative EMG in botulinum toxin treatment of cervical dystonia. A double-blind, placebo-controlled study. Ostergaard L et al. Electroencephalogr Clin Neurophysiol. 1994; 93: 434 – 9

Effects of local injections of botulinum toxin on electrophysiological parameters in patients with hemifacial spasm: role of synaptic activity and size of motor units. Glocker FX et al. Neurosci Lett. 1995; 187: 161 – 4

Short-term electrical stimulation enhances the effectiveness of Botulinum toxin in the treatment of lower limb spasticity in hemiparetic patients. Hesse S et al. Neurosci Lett. 1995; 201: 37 – 40

Physiological effects produced by botulinum toxin treatment of upper limb dystonia. Changes in reciprocal inhibition between forearm muscles. Priori A et al. Brain. 1995; 118 (Pt 3): 801 – 7

Electrophysiological studies in patients with blepharospasm before and after botulinum toxin A therapy. Behari M, Raju GB. J Neurol Sci. 1996; 135: 74 – 7

Unilateral injection of botulinum toxin in blepharospasm: single fiber electromyography and blink reflex study. Girlanda P et al. Mov Disord. 1996; 11: 27 – 31

Automated analysis of electromyographic (EMG) recordings during botulinum injections. Hunter DG et al. J Pediatr Ophthalmol Strabismus 1996; 33: 241 – 6

The variability in the clinical effect induced by botulinum toxin type A: the role of muscle activity in humans. Eleopra R et al. Mov Disord. 1997; 12: 89 – 94

The mechanism of action of botulinum toxin type A in focal dystonia is most probably through its dual effect on efferent (motor) and afferent pathways at the injected site. Giladi N. J Neurol Sci. 1997; 152: 132 – 5

Botulinum toxin in upper limb spasticity: study of reciprocal inhibition between forearm muscles. Girlanda P et al. Neuroreport 1997; 8: 3039 – 44

The EBD test–a clinical test for the detection of antibodies to botulinum toxin type A. Kessler KR, Benecke R. Mov Disord. 1997; 12: 95 – 9

Effects of botulinum neurotoxin type A on abducens motoneurons in the cat: alterations of the discharge pattern. Moreno-Lopez B et al. Neuroscience 1997; 81: 437 – 55

The corticomotor representation of upper limb muscles in writer's cramp and changes following botulinum toxin injection. Byrnes MI et al. Brain 1998; 121: 977–88

Sensory modulation of the blink reflex in patients with blepharospasm. Gomez-Wong E et al. J Arch Neurol. 1998; 55 : 1233–7

A re-evaluation of the mechanism of action of botulinum toxin on facial movement disorders in man. Leon F et al. Med Hypotheses 1998; 51: 305–7

Electromyographic quantification of the paralysing effect of botulinum toxin. Dressler D, Rothwell JC. Eur Neurol. 2000; 43 : 13–6

1.3   Pharmacological Studies

Properties and use of botulinum toxin and other microbial neurotoxins in medicine. Schantz EJ, Johnson EA. Microbiol Rev. 1992; 56: 80–99

Botulinum toxin type A purified neurotoxin complex for the treatment of blepharospasm: a dose-response study measuring eyelid force. Iwashige H et al. Jpn J Ophthalmol. 1995; 39: 424–31

The median paralysis unit: a more pharmacologically relevant unit of biologic activity for botulinum toxin. Pearce LB et al. Toxicon 1995; 33: 217–27

Reconstituted botulinum toxin type A does not lose potency in humans if it is refrozen or refrigerated for 2 weeks before use. Sloop RR et al. Neurology 1997; 48: 249–53

1.4   Molecular Biological Studies

SNAP-25 and syntaxin, but not synaptobrevin 2, cooperate in the regulated release of nerve growth factor. Blochl A. Neuroreport 1998; 9: 1701–5

Gangliosides are the binding substances in neural cells for tetanus and botulinum toxins in mice. Kitamura M et al. Biochim Biophys Acta 1999; 1441: 1–3

Functional characterisation of tetanus and botulinum neurotoxins binding domains. Lalli G et al. J Cell Sci. 1999; 112 (Pt 16): 2715–24

2   Side Effects

Distant effects of local injection of botulinum toxin [published erratum appears in Muscle Nerve 1988; 11 : 520] Lange DJ et al. Muscle Nerve 1987; 10: 552–5

Botulinum A toxin for the treatment of spasmodic torticollis: dysphagia and regional toxin spread. Borodic GE et al. Head Neck 1990; 12: 392–9

Acute angle-closure glaucoma following botulinum toxin injection for blepharospasm [see comments] Corridan P et al. Br J Ophthalmol. 1990; 74: 309–10

Polyradiculoneuritis following botulinum toxin therapy. Haug BA et al. J Neurol. 1990; 237: 62–3

Distant effects of locally injected botulinum toxin: a double-blind study of single fiber EMG changes [see comments] Lange DJ et al. Muscle Nerve 1991; 14: 672–5

Dysphagia after botulinum toxin injections for spasmodic torticollis: clinical and radiologic findings. Comella CL et al. Neurology 1992; 42: 1307–10

A comparative study of tear secretion in blepharospasm and hemifacial spasm patients treated with botulinum toxin. Price J, O'Day J. J Clin Neuroophthalmol. 1993; 13: 67–71

Localised autonomic failure due to botulinum toxin injection [see comments] Mann AC. J Neurol Neurosurg Psychiatry. 1994; 57: 1320

Botulinum toxin: influence on respiratory heart rate variation. Claus D et al. Mov Disord. 1995; 10: 574–9

Perianal thrombosis following injection therapy into the external anal sphincter using botulin toxin [letter] Jost WH et al. Dis Colon Rectum 1995; 38: 781

[Increased residual urine volume after local injection of botulinum A toxin]. Schnider P et al. Nervenarzt 1995; 66: 465–7

Pain and remote weakness in limbs injected with botulinum toxin A for writer's cramp. Sheean GL et al. Lancet. 1995; 346: 154–6

The swallowing side effects of botulinum toxin type A injection in spasmodic dysphonia. Holzer SE, Ludlow CL. Laryngoscope 1996; 106: 86–92

Development of general weakness in a patient with amyotrophic lateral sclerosis after focal botulinum toxin injection. Mezaki T et al. Neurology 1996; 46: 845–6

No effects on heart-rate variability and cardiovascular reflex tests after botulinum toxin treatment of cervical dystonia [letter]. Nebe A et al. Mov Disord. 1996; 11: 337–9

Generalised botulism-like syndrome after intramuscular injections of botulinum toxin type A: a report of two cases [letter]. Bakheit AM et al. J Neurol Neurosurg Psychiatry 1997; 62: 198

The swallowing side effects of botulinum toxin type A injection in spasmodic dysphonia. Buchholz DW, Neumann S. Dysphagia 1997; 12: 59–60

Idiosyncratic adverse reactions to intramuscular botulinum toxin type A injection. LeWitt PA, Trosch RM. Mov Disord. 1997; 12: 1064–7

Treatment of occupational cramp with botulinum toxin: diffusion of toxin to adjacent noninjected muscles. Ross MH et al. Muscle Nerve 1997; 20: 593–8

Brachial plexus neuropathy after botulinum toxin injection. Tarsy D. Neurology 1997; 49: 1176–7

Myasthenic crisis after botulinum toxin. Borodic G. Lancet 1998; 352: 1832

Necrotising fasciitis as a complication of botulinum toxin injection. Latimer PR et al. Eye 1998; 12: 51–3

Complications of botulinum A exotoxin for hyperfunctional lines. Matarasso SL. Int J Dermatol. 1999; 38: 641–55

3   Therapy Failure

Negative antibody response to long-term treatment of facial spasm with botulinum toxin. Gonnering RS. Am J Ophthalmol. 1988; 105: 313–5

Botulinum A toxin injection. Failures in clinical practice and a biomechanical system for the study of toxin-induced paralysis. Holds JB et al. Ophthal Plast Reconstr Surg. 1990; 6: 252–9

Botulinum antibodies in dystonic patients treated with type A botulinum toxin: frequency and significance [see comments] Zuber M et al. Neurology. 1993; 43: 1715–8

Oculinum injection-resistant blepharospasm in young patients. Gausas RE et al. Ophthal Plast Reconstr Surg. 1994; 10: 193

Antibodies to botulinum toxin [letter; comment]. Borodic GE et al. Neurology 1995; 45: 204

Response and immunoresistance to botulinum toxin injections. Jankovic J, Schwartz K. Neurology 1995; 45: 1743–6

Botulinum toxin therapy, immunologic resistance, and problems with available materials. Borodic G et al. Neurology 1996; 46: 26–9

Sensitive assay for measurement of antibodies to Clostridium botulinum neurotoxins A, B, and E: use of hapten-labeled-antibody elution to isolate specific complexes. Doellgast GJ et al. J Infect Dis. 1997; 175: 633–7

Botulinum toxin therapy failure: causes, evaluation procedures and management strategies. Dressler D. Eur J Neurol. 1997; 4/suppl 2: S67–S70

Endogenous antibody production to botulinum toxin in an adult with intestinal colonization botulism and underlying Crohn's disease. Griffin PM et al. Neurology 1997; 49: 701–7

Botulinum A toxin therapy: neutralizing and nonneutralizing antibodies–therapeutic consequences. Goschel H et al. Exp Neurol. 1997; 147: 96–102

Mouse bioassay versus Western blot assay for botulinum toxin antibodies: correlation with clinical response. Hanna PA, Jankovic J Neurology 1998 Jun;50(6):1624–9

Depletion of neutralising antibodies resensitises a secondary non-responder to botulinum A neurotoxin. Naumann M et al. J Neurol Neurosurg Psychiatry 1998; 65: 924–7

A radioimmuno-precipitation assay for antibodies to botulinum A. Palace J et al. Neurology 1998; 50: 1463–6

Variability of the immunologic and clinical response in dystonic patients immunoresistant to botulinum toxin injections. Sankhla C et al. Mov Disord. 1998; 13: 150–4

Comparison of mouse bioassay and immunoprecipitation assay for botulinum toxin antibodies. Hanna PA et al. J Neurol Neurosurg Psychiatry 1999; 66: 612–6

4 Non-A Botulinum Toxins

Therapeutic use of type F botulinum toxin [letter]. Ludlow CL et al. N Engl J Med. 1992; 326: 349–50

Use of botulinum toxin type F injections to treat torticollis in patients with immunity to botulinum toxin type A. Greene PE, Fahn S. Mov Disord. 1993; 8: 479–83

Optimisation of botulinum treatment for cervical and axial dystonias: experience with a Japanese type A toxin. Mezaki T et al. J Neurol Neurosurg Psychiatry 1994; 57: 1535–7

Comparison of therapeutic efficacies of type A and F botulinum toxins for blephar-ospasm: a double-blind, controlled study. Mezaki T et al. Neurology 1995; 45: 506–8

Botulinum toxin F in the treatment of torticollis clinically resistant to botulinum toxin A. Sheean GL, Lees AJ. J Neurol Neurosurg Psychiatry 1995; 59: 601–7

Botulinum toxin type B in the treatment of cervical dystonia: a pilot study. Tsui JK et al. Neurology 1995; 45: 2109–10

Response to botulinum toxin F in seronegative botulinum toxin A–resistant pa-tients. Greene PE, Fahn S. Mov-Disord. 1996; 11: 181–4

Safety and efficacy of NeuroBloc (botulinum toxin type B) in type A-responsive cervical dystonia. Brashear A et al. Mov Disord. 1997; 12: 772–5

Botulinum toxin type B: a double-blind, placebo-controlled, safety and efficacy study in cervical dystonia. Lew MF et al. Neurology 1997; 49: 701–7

Human response to botulinum toxin injection: type B compared with type A. Sloop RR et al. Neurology 1997; 49: 189–94

BotB (botulinum toxin type B): evaluation of safety and tolerability in botulinum toxin type A-resistant cervical dystonia patients (preliminary study). Truong DD et al. J Clin Microbiol. 1997; 35: 578–83

Further studies using higher doses of botulinum toxin type F for torticollis resist-ant to botulinum toxin type A. Houser MK et al. Neurology 1998; 51: 1494–6

Safety and efficacy of NeuroBloc (botulinum toxin type B) in type A-resistant cer-vical dystonia. Brin MF et al. Neurology 1999; 53: 1431–8

Botulinum toxin type F for treatment of dystonia: long-term experience. Chen R et al. Neurology 1999; 53: 1439–46

5   Potency Comparison

Dose standardisation of botulinum toxin [letter]. Schantz EJ, Johnson EA. Lancet 1990; 335: 421

Potency of frozen/thawed botulinum toxin type A in the treatment of torsion dys-tonia [letter; comment]. Greene P. Otolaryngol Head Neck Surg. 1993; 109: 968–9

Dose standardisation of botulinum toxin [letter; comment]. Pickett AM, Hamble-ton P. Lancet 1994; 344: 474–5

Botulinum toxin potency: a mystery resolved by the median paralysis [letter; com-ment]. Pearce LB et al. J R Soc Med. 1994; 87: 571–2

Dose standardisation of botulinum toxin [letter]. Marion MH et al. J Neurol Neuro-surg Psychiatry 1995; 59: 102–3

The median paralysis unit: a more pharmacologically relevant unit of biologic ac-tivity for botulinum toxin. Pearce LB et al. Toxicon 1995; 33: 217–27

Botulinum A toxins: units versus units. Wohlfarth K et al. Naunyn-Schmiedebergs Arch Pharmacol. 1997; 355: 335–40

DYSBOT: a single-blind, randomized parallel study to determine whether any dif-ferences can be detected in the efficacy and tolerability of two formulations of botulinum toxin type A–Dysport and Botox–assuming a ratio of 4 : 1. Sampaio C et al. Mov Disord. 1997; 12: 1013–8

Comparing biological potencies of Botox and Dysport with a mouse diaphragm model may mislead. Dressler D et al. J Neurol Neurosurg Psychiatry 1998; 64: 6–12

Dose standardization of botulinum toxin. Krack P et al. J Neurol. 1998; 245: 332; Mov Disord. 1998; 13: 749–51

A double blind, randomised, parallel group study to investigate the dose equivalence of Dysport and Botox in the treatment of cervical dystonia. Odergren T et al. J Neurol Neurosurg Psychiatry 1998: 64; 6–12

II Clinical Applications

1 Reviews

1.1 Consensus Statements

Botulinum toxin therapy of eye muscle disorders. Safety and effectiveness. American Academy of Ophthalmology. Ophthalmology 1989; Pt 2: 37–41

Botulinum toxin. Consens-Statement 1990 Nov 12–14; 8(8): 1–20

Assessment: the clinical usefulness of botulinum toxin-A in treating neurologic disorders. Report of the Therapeutics and Technology Assessment Subcommittee of the American Academy of Neurology. Neurology 1990; 40: 1332–6

Consensus panel considers uses of botulinum toxin. Clin Pharm. 1991; 10: 88

Consensus conference. Clinical use of botulinum toxin. National Institutes of Health. Conn Med. 1991; 55: 471–7

Clinical use of botulinum toxin. National Institutes of Health Consensus Development Conference Statement, November 12–14, 1990. Arch Neurol. 1991; 48: 1294–8

Consensus statement on physician training for the treatment of dystonia with botulinum toxin. The Canadian Movement Disorders Group. Can J Neurol Sci. 1992; 19: 522

Consensus statement for the management of focal dystonias. Williams A. Br J Hosp Med. 1993; 50: 655–9

Training guidelines for the use of botulinum toxin for the treatment of neurologic disorders. Report of the Therapeutics and Technology Assessment Subcommittee of the American Academy of Neurology. Neurology 1994; 44: 2401–3

Guidelines for the therapeutic use of botulinum toxin in movement disorders. Italian Study Group for Movement Disorders, Italian Society of Neurology. Berardelli A et al. Ital J Neurol Sci. 1997; 18: 261–9

1.2 General

Botulinum toxin: the story of its development for the treatment of human disease. Schantz EJ, Johnson EA. Perspect Biol Med. 1997; 40: 317–27

One man's poison–clinical applications of botulinum toxin. Hallett M. N Engl J Med. 1999; 341: 118–20

1.3 History

Historical note on the therapeutic use of botulinum toxin in neurological disorders. Erbguth FJ. J Neurol Neurosurg Psychiatry 1996; 60: 151

Historical aspects of botulinum toxin: Justinus Kerner (1786 – 1862) and the "sausage poison". Erbguth FJ, Naumann M. Neurology 1999; 53: 1850 – 3

1.4 Neurology

Neurological application of botulinum toxin. Kumar P, Crowley WJ Jr. Mo Med. 1989; 86: 815 – 7

Botulinum toxin and dystonias. Drug Ther Bull. 1991; 29: 102 – 3

Interventional neurology: treatment of neurological conditions with local injection of botulinum toxin. Brin MF. Arch Neurobiol Madr. 1991; 54: 173 – 89

Botulinum toxin therapy for neurologic disorders. Tim R, Massey JM. Postgrad Med. 1992; 91: 327 – 32, 334

Botulinum toxin in the treatment of neurological disorders. Denislic M et al. Ann NY Acad Sci. 1994; 710: 76 – 87

Botulinum toxin in movement disorders. Jankovic J. Curr Opin Neurol. 1994; 7: 358 – 66

Botulinum toxin in the cerebral palsies. Neville B. BMJ. 1994; 309: 1526 – 7

Botulinum toxin treatment in clinical neurology. Van den Bergh P. Acta Neurol Belg. 1995; 95: 70 – 9

1.5 Ophthalmology

Botulinum-A toxin for ocular muscle disorders. Lancet 1986; 1: 76 – 7

Botulinum-A toxin for ocular muscle disorders [letter]. Elston JS. Lancet 1986; 1: 265 – 6

Botulinum-A toxin for ocular muscle disorders [letter]. Spector JG, Burde RM. Lancet 1986; 1: 855

Botulinum toxin in ophthalmology. Dunlop D et al. Aust NZ J Ophthalmol. 1988; 16: 15 – 20

Botulinum toxin for ocular muscle disorders. Med Lett Drugs Ther. 1990; 32: 100 – 2

Botulinum A toxin (Oculinum) in ophthalmology. Osako M, Keltner JL. Surv Ophthalmol. 1991; 36: 28 – 46

The current use of botulinum toxin therapy in strabismus. Rosenbaum AL. Arch Ophthalmol. 1996; 114: 213 – 4

1.6 Gastroenterology

Review article: the use of botulinum toxin in the alimentary tract. Albanese A et al. Aliment Pharmacol Ther. 1995; 9: 599 – 604

Treatment of achalasia–whalebone to botulinum toxin [editorial; comment]. Cohen S, Parkman HP. N Engl J Med. 1995; 332: 815 – 6

Botulinum toxin: a new therapeutic use. Ogilvie J et al. Gastroenterol Nurs. 1995; 18: 92 – 5

Knife, balloon, drugs, and now the needle for treatment of achalasia cardia [editorial; comment]. Bhatia SJ, Aggarwal R. Indian J Gastroenterol. 1996; 15: 82 – 5

Botulinum toxin for achalasia: to be or not to be? [comment]. Castell DO, Katzka
  DA. Gastroenterology 1996; 110: 1650 – 2

1.7 Otorhinolaryngology

Treatment of speech and voice disorders with botulinum toxin. Ludlow CL. JAMA.
  1990; 264: 2671 – 5

2 Dystonia

2.1 Cranial Dystonia

2.1.1 Blepharospasm, Meige Syndrome

Treatment of blepharospasm with botulinum toxin. A preliminary report. Frueh BR
  et al. Arch Ophthalmol. 1984; 102: 1464 – 8
Effect of treatment with botulinum toxin on neurogenic blepharospasm. Elston JS,
  Russell RW. Br Med J Clin Res Ed. 1985; 290: 1857 – 9
Management of blepharospasm. Kennedy RH et al. Ophthal Plast Reconstr Surg.
  1985; 1: 253 – 61
Blepharospasm, Meige syndrome, and hemifacial spasm: treatment with botuli-
  num toxin. Mauriello JA Jr. Neurology 1985; 35: 1499 – 500
The use of botulinum toxin in blepharospasm. Shorr N et al. Am J Ophthalmol.
  1985; 99: 542 – 6
Treatment of blepharospasm with botulinum toxin. Tsoy EA et al. Am J Ophthal-
  mol. 1985; 99: 176 – 9
Treatment of facial spasm with Oculinum (C botulinum toxin). Biglan AW, May M. J
  Pediatr Ophthalmol Strabismus. 1986; 23: 216 – 21
Botulinum toxin in the management of blepharospasm. Dutton JJ, Buckley EG.
  Arch Neurol. 1986; 43: 380 – 2
Treatment of facial spasm with botulinum toxin. An interim report. Frueh BR,
  Musch-DC. Ophthalmology 1986; 93: 917 – 23
The use of botulinum toxin in the medical management of benign essential ble-
  pharospasm. Perman KI et al. Ophthalmology 1986; 93: 1 – 3
Botulinum toxin for the treatment of essential blepharospasm. Shore JW et al.
  Ophthalmic Surg. 1986; 17: 747 – 53
Treatment of blepharospasm with medication, surgery and type A botulinum tox-
  in. Arthurs B et al. Can J Ophthalmol. 1987; 22: 24 – 8
Benign essential blepharospasm treated with botulinum toxin. Berlin AJ et al.
  Cleve Clin J Med. 1987; 54: 421 – 6
Botulinum toxin for benign essential blepharospasm, hemifacial spasm and age-
  related lower eyelid entropion. Carruthers J, Stubbs HA. Can J Neurol Sci. 1987;
  14: 42 – 5
Long-term results of treatment of idiopathic blepharospasm with botulinum toxin
  injections. Elston JS. Br J Ophthalmol. 1987; 71: 664 – 8
Effectiveness of botulinum toxin therapy for essential blepharospasm. Engstrom
  PF et al. Ophthalmology 1987; 94: 971 – 5
Treatment of blepharospasm with high dose brow injection of botulinum toxin.
  Kristan RW, Stasior OG. Ophthal Plast Reconstr Surg. 1987; 3: 25 – 7

Use of botulinum toxin in the treatment of one hundred patients with facial dyskinesias. Mauriello JA Jr et al. Ophthalmology 1987; 94: 976 – 9

Use of botulinum toxin in blepharospasm and other facial spasms. Ruusuvaara P, Setala K. Acta Ophthalmol Copenh. 1987; 65: 313 – 9

Management of facial spasm with Clostridium botulinum toxin, type A (Oculinum) [see comments]. Biglan AW et al. Arch Otolaryngol Head Neck Surg. 1988; 114: 1407 – 12

Botulinum toxin treatment of blepharospasm. Elston JS. Adv Neurol. 1988; 50: 579 – 81

The effect of omitting botulinum toxin from the lower eyelid in blepharospasm treatment. Frueh-BR et al. Am J Ophthalmol. 1988; 106: 45 – 7

Botulinum toxin injections in the treatment of blepharospasm, hemifacial spasm, and eyelid fasciculations. Kraft SP; Lang AE. Can J Neurol Sci. 1988; 15: 276 – 80

Use of botulinum toxin in Meige's disease. Maurri S et al. Riv Neurol. 1988; 58: 245 – 8

Blepharospasm and its treatment, with emphasis on the use of botulinum toxin. Borodic GE, Cozzolino D. Plast Reconstr Surg. 1989; 83: 546 – 54

[Botulinum toxin in therapy of craniocervical dystonia]. Dressler-D et al. Nervenarzt 1989; 60: 386 – 93

Essential blepharospasm and related dystonias. Jordan DR et al. Surv Ophthalmol. 1989; 34: 123 – 32

Treatment of blepharospasm with botulinum toxin. Kennedy RH et al. Mayo Clin Proc. 1989; 64: 1085 – 90

Botulinum A toxin treatment for eyelid spasm, spasmodic torticollis and apraxia of eyelid opening. Defazio G et al. Ital J Neurol Sci. 1990; 11: 275 – 80

Eyelid movements before and after botulinum therapy in patients with lid spasm. Manning KA et al. Ann Neurol. 1990; 28: 653 – 60

Botulinum toxin for the treatment of blepharospasm and strabismus. Paul TO. West J Med. 1990; 153: 187

Long-term treatment of involuntary facial spasms using botulinum toxin. Ruusuvaara P, Setala K. Acta Ophthalmol Copenh. 1990; 68: 331 – 8

A five-year analysis of botulinum toxin type A injections: some unusual features. Balkan RJ, Poole T. Ann Ophthalmol. 1991; 23: 326 – 33

Botulinum toxin in the treatment of facial dyskinesias. Chong PN et al. Ann Acad Med Singapore 1991; 20: 223 – 7

Natural history of treatment of facial dyskinesias with botulinum toxin: a study of 50 consecutive patients over seven years. Mauriello JA, Aljian J. Br J Ophthalmol. 1991; 75: 737 – 9

Treatment of blepharospasm and hemifacial spasm with botulinum A toxin: a Canadian multicentre study. Taylor JD et al. Can J Ophthalmol. 1991; 26: 133 – 8

Botulinum toxin injections for treatment of blepharospasm and hemifacial spasm. Wirtschafter JD, Rubenfeld M. Int Ophthalmol Clin. 1991; 31: 117 – 32

The management of blepharospasm and hemifacial spasm. Elston JS. J Neurol. 1992; 239: 5 – 8

Frontalis suspension for essential blepharospasm unresponsive to botulinum toxin therapy. First results. Roggenkamper P, Nussgens Z. Ger J Ophthalmol. 1993; 2: 426 – 8

Botulinum toxin treatment in patients with focal dystonia and hemifacial spasm. A multicenter study of the Italian Movement Disorder Group. Berardelli A et al. Ital J Neurol Sci. 1993; 14: 361 – 7

Abnormal eye movements in blepharospasm and involuntary levator palpebrae inhibition. Clinical and pathophysiological considerations. Aramideh M et al. Brain 1994; 117: 1457 – 74

Electromyographic features of levator palpebrae superioris and orbicularis oculi muscles in blepharospasm. Aramideh M et al. Brain 1994; 117: 27 – 38

Botulinum toxin therapy for blepharospasm in the otolaryngology clinic. Lassen LF, Adams J. ORL Head Neck Nurs. 1994; 12: 12 – 3

Efficacy and side effects of botulinum toxin treatment for blepharospasm and hemifacial spasm. Price J, O'Day J. Aust NZ J Ophthalmol. 1994; 22: 255 – 60

Pretarsal application of botulinum toxin for treatment of blepharospasm [see comments] Aramideh M et al. J Neurol Neurosurg Psychiatry. 1995; 59: 309 – 11

Botulinum toxin type A purified neurotoxin complex for the treatment of blepharospasm: a dose-response study measuring eyelid force. Iwashige H et al. Jpn J Ophthalmol. 1995; 39: 424 – 31

Long-term treatment of blepharospasm with botulinum toxin type A. Nussgens Z, Roggenkamper P. Ger J Ophthalmol. 1995; 4: 363 – 7

Pretarsal injections of botulinum toxin improve blepharospasm in previously unresponsive patients [letter]. Albanese A et al. J Neurol Neurosurg Psychiatry 1996; 60: 693 – 4

Botulinum-A toxin in the treatment of craniocervical muscle spasms: short- and long-term, local and systemic effects. Dutton JJ. Surv Ophthalmol. 1996; 41: 51 – 65

Treatment selections of 239 patients with blepharospasm and Meige syndrome over 11 years. Mauriello JA Jr et al. Br J Ophthalmol. 1996; 80: 1073 – 6

Pretarsal injections of botulinum toxin improve blephospasm in previously unresponsive patients. Kowal L. J Neurol Neurosurg Psychiatry 1997; 63: 556

Comparison of two botulinum-toxin preparations in the treatment of essential blepharospasm. Nussgens Z, Roggenkamper P. Graefes Arch Clin Exp Ophthalmol. 1997; 235: 197 – 9

Botulinum A toxin treatment for blepharospasm and Meige syndrome: report of 100 patients. Poungvarin N et al. J Med Assoc Thai. 1997; 80: 1 – 8

Frontalis suspension in the treatment of essential blepharospasm unresponsive to botulinum-toxin therapy: long-term results. Roggenkamper P, Nussgens Z. Graefes Arch Clin Exp Ophthalmol 1997; 235: 486 – 9

Oculinum injection-resistant blepharospasm in young patients. Roggenkamper P, Nussgens Z. Ophthal Plast Reconstr Surg. 1997; 13: 73

2.1.2 Apraxia of Eyelid Opening

Botulinum A toxin treatment for eyelid spasm, spasmodic torticollis and apraxia of eyelid opening. Defazio G et al. Ital J Neurol Sci. 1990; 11: 275 – 80

Frontalis suspension for essential blepharospasm unresponsive to botulinum toxin therapy. First results. Roggenkamper P, Nussgens Z. Ger J Ophthalmol. 1993; 2: 426 – 8

Botulinum A toxin for the so-called apraxia of lid opening. Lepore-V et al. Mov-Disord. 1995 Jul; 10(4): 525 – 6

Pretarsal injection of botulinum toxin for blepharospasm and apraxia of eyelid opening [letter; comment]. Comment on: J Neurol Neurosurg Psychiatry 1995; 59: 309 – 11 Jankovic J. J Neurol Neurosurg Psychiatry 1996; 60: 704

Botulinum toxin treatment of apraxia of eyelid opening in progressive supranuclear palsy: report of two cases. Piccione F et al. Arch Phys Med Rehabil. 1997; 78: 525 – 9

2.1.3   Mandibular Dystonia

Treatment of oromandibular dystonia with botulinum toxin. Hermanowicz N, Truong DD. Laryngoscope 1991; 101: 1216 – 8

Oromandibular dystonia treated with botulinum toxin: report of case. Heise GJ, Mullen MP. J Oral Maxillofac Surg. 1995; 53: 332 – 5; discussion

Auctioneer's jaw: a case of occupational oromandibular hemidystonia. Scolding NJ, Lees AJ. Mov Disord. 1995; 10: 508 – 9

Bruxism after brain injury: successful treatment with botulinum toxin-A. Ivanhoe CB et al. Arch Phys Med Rehabil. 1997; 78: 1272 – 3

Botulinum toxin A in patients with oromandibular dystonia: long-term follow-up. Tan EK, Jankovic J. Neurology 1999; 53: 2102 – 7

2.1.4   Tongue Dystonia

Botulinum toxin injections for lingual dystonia [letter]. Blitzer A et al. Laryngoscope 1991; 101: 799

2.2   Cervical Dystonia

A pilot study on the use of botulinum toxin in spasmodic torticollis. Tsui JK et al. Can J Neurol Sci. 1985; 12: 314 – 6

Double-blind study of botulinum toxin in spasmodic torticollis. Tsui JK et al. Lancet. 1986; 2: 245 – 7

Botulinum toxin for correction of torticollis. Ben-Ezra D et al. Bull Soc Belge Ophtalmol. 1987; 221/222: 295 – 301

Local treatment of spasmodic torticollis with botulinum toxin. Tsui JK et al. Can J Neurol Sci. 1987; 14 (3 Suppl): 533 – 5

Botulinum toxin treatment of spasmodic torticollis [letter]. Stell R et al. BMJ. 1988; 297: 616

Botulinum toxin in cervical dystonia. Tsui JK, Calne DB. Adv Neurol. 1988; 49: 473 – 8

[Botulinum toxin in therapy of craniocervical dystonia]. Dressler D et al. Nervenarzt 1989; 60: 386 – 93

Controlled trial of botulinum toxin injections in the treatment of spasmodic torticollis [see comments]. Gelb DJ et al. Neurology 1989; 39: 80 – 4

Botulinum toxin in torticollis [letter; comment]. Stell R et al. Neurology 1989; 39: 1403 – 4

Botulinum A toxin treatment for eyelid spasm, spasmodic torticollis and apraxia of eyelid opening. Defazio G et al. Ital J Neurol Sci. 1990; 11: 275 – 80

Double-blind, placebo-controlled trial of botulinum toxin injections for the treatment of spasmodic torticollis. Greene P et al. Neurology 1990; 40: 1213 – 8

Botulinum toxin injections for cervical dystonia. Jankovic J, Schwartz K. Neurology 1990; 40: 277 – 80

Failure of fixed-dose, fixed muscle injection of botulinum toxin in torticollis. Koller W et al. Clin-Neuropharmacol. 1990; 13: 355 – 8

Treatment of idiopathic spasmodic torticollis with botulinum-A toxin: a pilot study of 19 patients. Lorentz IT et al. Med J Aust. 1990; 152: 528 – 30

Botulinum toxin treatment of spasmodic torticollis. Davies L, Lorentz IT. Clin Exp Neurol. 1991; 28: 197 – 8

Low dose botulinum toxin in spasmodic torticollis [see comments]. D'Costa DF, Abbott RJ. J R Soc Med. 1991; 84: 650 – 1

Electromyographic guidance of botulinum toxin treatment in cervical dystonia. Dubinsky RM et al. Clin Neuropharmacol. 1991; 14: 262 – 7

Treatment of spasmodic torticollis with local injections of botulinum toxin. One-year follow-up in 37 patients. Poewe W et al. J Neurol. 1992; 239: 21 – 5

Botulinum toxin treatment of spasmodic torticollis [see comments]. Anderson TJ et al. J R Soc Med. 1992; 85: 524 – 9

Botulinum toxin injection for spasmodic torticollis: increased magnitude of benefit with electromyographic assistance. Comella CL et al. Neurology 1992; 42: 878 – 82

Treatment of cervical dystonia hand spasms and laryngeal dystonia with botulinum toxin. Lees AJ et al. J Neurol. 1992; 239: 1 – 4

Low dose botulinum toxin for spasmodic torticollis [letter; comment]. Moore AP. J R Soc Med. 1992; 85(5): 304

Local treatment of dystonia and spasticity with injections of botulinum-A toxin. Calne S. Axone 1993; 14: 85 – 8

Botulinum toxin treatment in patients with focal dystonia and hemifacial spasm. A multicenter study of the Italian Movement Disorder Group. Berardelli A et al. Ital J Neurol Sci. 1993; 14: 361 – 7

Use of botulinum toxin in the treatment of cervical dystonia. Poewe W, Wissel J. Baillieres Clin Neurol. 1993; 2: 179 – 85

Efficacy of botulinum toxin for cervical dystonia. A comparison of methods for evaluation. Odergren T et al. Scand J Rehabil Med. 1994; 26: 191 – 5

Botulinum toxin in cervical dystonia: low dosage with electromyographic guidance. Brans JW et al. J Neurol. 1995; 242: 529 – 34

Double-blind, placebo-controlled study of botulinum toxin injections in the treatment of cervical dystonia. Lu CS et al. J Formos Med Assoc. 1995; 94: 189 – 92

Botulinum-A toxin in the treatment of craniocervical muscle spasms: short- and long-term, local and systemic effects. Dutton JJ. Surv Ophthalmol. 1996; 41: 51 – 65

Spasmodic torticollis: a case report and review of therapies. Smith DL, DeMario MC. J Am Board Fam Pract. 1996; 9: 435 – 41

Severe and prolonged dysphagia complicating botulinum toxin A injections for dystonia in Machado-Joseph disease. Tuite PJ, Lang AE. Neurology 1996; 46: 846

Long-term treatment of cervical dystonia with botulinum toxin A: efficacy, safety, and antibody frequency. German Dystonia Study Group. Kessler KR et al. Neurol Neurosurg Psychiatry 1998;64: 577 – 80

What is the optimal dose of botulinum toxin A in the treatment of cervical dystonia? Results of a double blind, placebo controlled, dose ranging study using Dysport. German Dystonia Study Group. Poewe W et al. Neurol Neurosurg Psychiatry 1998;64: 13 – 7

Painful cervical dystonia: clinical features and response to treatment with botulinum toxin. Tarsy D, First ER. Mov Disord. 1999; 14: 1043 – 5

2.3 Laryngeal Dystonia

2.3.1 Voice Triggered Laryngeal Dystonia

2.3.1.1 Spasmodic Dysphonia/Adductor Type

Botulinum toxin (BOTOX) for the treatment of "spastic dysphonia" as part of a trial of toxin injections for the treatment of other cranial dystonias [letter]. Blitzer A et al. Laryngoscope 1986; 96: 1300 – 1

Botulinum toxin for relief of spasmodic dysphonia [letter]. Gacek RR. Arch Otolaryngol Head Neck Surg. 1987; 113: 1240

Botulinum toxin injection of the vocal fold for spasmodic dysphonia. A preliminary report. Miller RH et al. Arch Otolaryngol Head Neck Surg. 1987; 113: 603 – 5

Localized injections of botulinum toxin for the treatment of focal laryngeal dystonia (spastic dysphonia). Blitzer A et al. Laryngoscope 1988; 98: 193 – 7

Effects of botulinum toxin injections on speech in adductor spasmodic dysphonia. Ludlow CL et al. Neurology 1988; 38: 1220 – 5

Adductor laryngeal dystonia (spastic dysphonia): treatment with local injections of botulinum toxin (Botox). Brin MF et al. Mov-Disord. 1989; 4: 287 – 96

Indirect laryngoscopic approach for injection of botulinum toxin in spasmodic dysphonia. Ford CN et al. Otolaryngol Head Neck Surg. 1990; 103: 752 – 8

Spasmodic dysphonia: botulinum toxin injection after recurrent nerve surgery. Ludlow CL et al. Otolaryngol Head Neck Surg. 1990; 102: 122 – 31

Laryngeal dystonia: a series with botulinum toxin therapy. Blitzer A, Brin MF. Ann Otol Rhinol Laryngol. 1991; 100: 85 – 9

Double-blind controlled study of botulinum toxin in adductor spasmodic dysphonia. Truong DD et al. Laryngoscope 1991; 101: 630 – 4

Treatment of cervical dystonia hand spasms and laryngeal dystonia with botulinum toxin. Lees AJ et al. J Neurol. 1992; 239: 1 – 4

Effects of botulinum toxin therapy in patients with adductor spasmodic dysphonia: acoustic, aerodynamic, and videoendoscopic findings. Zwirner P et al. Laryngoscope 1992; 102: 400 – 6

Unilateral versus bilateral botulinum toxin injections in spasmodic dysphonia: acoustic and perceptual results. Adams SG et al. J Otolaryngol. 1993; 22: 171 – 5

Botulinum toxin injection for adductor spastic dysphonia: patient self-ratings of voice and phonatory effort after three successive injections. Aronson AE et al. Laryngoscope 1993; 103: 683 – 92

Botulinum toxin A for cricopharyngeal dystonia [letter]. Dunne J et al. Lancet. 1993; 342: 559

Spasmodic dysphonia and laryngeal botulinum toxin injection. Smith ME. West J Med. 1993; 159: 74

The use of botulinum toxin in the treatment of adductor spasmodic dysphonia. Whurr R et al. J Neurol Neurosurg Psychiatry 1993; 56: 526 – 30

Spasmodic dysphonia: new diagnosis and treatment opportunities. Cook MJ, Lewin JS. Nurse Pract. 1994; 19: 67 – 73

Adductor laryngeal breathing dystonia in a patient with lubag (X-linked dystonia-Parkinsonism syndrome). Lew MF et al. Mov Disord. 1994; 9: 318 – 20

A comparison of the efficacy of unilateral versus bilateral botulinum toxin injections in the treatment of adductor spasmodic dysphonia. Maloney AP, Morrison MD. J-Otolaryngol. 1994; 23: 160 – 4

Spasmodic dysphonia. Emotional status and botulinum toxin treatment. Murry T et al. Arch Otolaryngol Head Neck Surg. 1994; 120: 310 – 6

Technique for injection of botulinum toxin through the flexible nasolaryngoscope. Rhew K et al. Otolaryngol Head Neck Surg. 1994; 111: 787 – 94

Botulinum toxin in the treatment of adductor spasmodic dysphonia. Thompson AR. J Ark Med Soc. 1994; 90: 383 – 5

Measurement of laryngeal resistance in the evaluation of botulinum toxin injection for treatment of focal laryngeal dystonia. Witsell DL et al. Laryngoscope 1994; 104: 8 – 11

Comparison of botulinum toxin injection procedures in adductor spasmodic dysphonia. Adams SG et al. J Otolaryngol. 1995; 24: 345 – 51

Combined-modality treatment of adductor spasmodic dysphonia with botulinum toxin and voice therapy. Murry T, Woodson GE. J Voice 1995; 9: 460 – 5

Laryngeal image analysis following botulinum toxin injections in spasmodic dysphonia. Wong DL et al. J Otolaryngol. 1995; 24: 64 – 8

Effect of neuromuscular activity on the response to botulinum toxin injections in spasmodic dysphonia. Wong DL et al. J Otolaryngol. 1995; 24: 209 – 16

Effects of botulinum toxin type A injections on aerodynamic measures of spasmodic dysphonia. Adams SG et al. Laryngoscope 1996; 106: 296 – 300

Long-term effects of botulinum toxin injections in spasmodic dysphonia. Davidson BJ, Ludlow CL. Ann Otol Rhinol Laryngol. 1996; 105: 33 – 42

Longitudinal phonatory characteristics after botulinum toxin type A injection. Fisher KV et al. J Speech Hear Res. 1996; 39: 968 – 80

Analysis of factors affecting botulinum toxin results in spasmodic dysphonia. Inagi K et al. J Voice 1996; 10: 306 – 313

Alternating unilateral botulinum toxin type A (BOTOX) injections for spasmodic dysphonia. Koriwchak MJ et al. Laryngoscope 1996; 106: 1476 – 81

Prospective study of patients' subjective responses to botulinum toxin injection for spasmodic dysphonia. Liu TC et al. J Otolaryngol. 1996; 25: 66 – 74

Correlation between clinical response and injection quality in treatment of spasmodic dysphonia. Tewary AK. J Laryngol Otol. 1996; 110: 551 – 3

Botulinum toxin management of spasmodic dysphonia (laryngeal dystonia): a 12-year experience in more than 900 patients. Blitzer A et al. Adv Neurol 1998; 78: 237 – 52

Laryngeal dystonia (spasmodic dysphonia): observations of 901 patients and treatment with botulinum toxin. Brin MF et al. Adv Neurol 1998; 78: 135 – 52

Botulinum toxin treatment for spasmodic dysphonia: percutaneous versus transoral approach. Garcia Ruiz PJ et al. J Clin Neuropharmacol. 1998; 21: 196 – 8

Unilateral versus bilateral botulinum toxin injections in adductor spasmodic dysphonia. Langeveld TP et al. Int J Lang Commun Disord 1998; 33 Suppl 327 – 9

Laryngeal chemodenervation: effects of injection site, dose, and volume. Lee P, Paniello RC. Laryngoscope 1998;108 : 1435 – 41

Meta-analysis of botulinum toxin treatment of spasmodic dysphonia: a review of 22studies. Whurr R et al. Ann Otol Rhinol Laryngol. 1999; 108: 1140 – 5

2.3.1.2 Spasmodic Dysphonia/Abductor Type

Laryngeal dystonia: a series with botulinum toxin therapy. Blitzer A, Brin MF. Ann Otol Rhinol Laryngol. 1991; 100: 85 – 9

A method for the treatment of abductor spasmodic dysphonia with botulinum toxin injections: a preliminary report. Rontal M et al. Laryngoscope 1991; 101: 911 – 4

Treatment of adductor laryngeal breathing dystonia with botulinum toxin type A. Grillone GA et al. Laryngoscope 1994; 104: 30 – 2

2.3.2 Non-Voice Triggered Laryngeal Dystonia

[Abnormal movements of the larynx. Diagnostic approach and therapeutic perspectives]. Angelard B et al. Ann Otolaryngol Chir Cervicofac. 1993; 110: 125 – 8

2.4 Limb Dystonia

2.4.1 Upper Extremities

Treatment of cervical dystonia hand spasms and laryngeal dystonia with botulinum toxin. Lees AJ et al. J Neurol. 1992; 239: 1 – 4

Botulinum toxin therapy for limb dystonias. Yoshimura DM et al. Neurology 1992; 42: 627 – 30

Use of botulinum toxin in the treatment of hand dystonia. Jankovic J, Schwartz KS. J Hand Surg Am. 1993; 18: 883 – 7

Writer's cramp–a focal dystonia: etiology, diagnosis, and treatment. Rhoad RC, Stern PJ. J Hand Surg Am. 1993; 18: 541 – 4

Botulinum toxin in the treatment of writer's cramp: a double-blind study. Tsui JK et al. Neurology 1993; 43: 183 – 5

Long-term botulinum toxin treatment of focal hand dystonia. Karp BI et al. Neurology 1994; 44: 70 – 6

Double-blind trial of botulinum toxin for treatment of focal hand dystonia. Cole R et al. Mov Disord. 1995; 10: 466 – 71

Pain and remote weakness in limbs injected with botulinum toxin A for writer's cramp. Sheean GL et al. Lancet 1995; 346: 154 – 6

Localizing muscles for botulinum toxin treatment of focal hand dystonia. Geenen C et al. Can J Neurol Sci. 1996; 23: 194 – 7

Approach to the treatment of limb disorders with botulinum toxin A. Experience with 187 patients. Pullman SL et al. Arch Neurol. 1996; 53: 617 – 24

Treatment of nonoccupational limb and trunk dystonia with botulinum toxin. Quirk JA et al. Mov Disord. 1996; 11: 377 – 83

Botulinum toxin in the treatment of writer's cramp. Turjanski N et al. Clin Neuropharmacol. 1996; 19: 314 – 20

Botulinum toxin in writer's cramp: objective response evaluation in 31 patients. Wissel J et al. J Neurol Neurosurg Psychiatry 1996; 61: 172 – 5

Treatment of occupational cramp with botulinum toxin: diffusion of toxin to adjacent noninjected muscles. Ross MH et al. Muscle Nerve 1997; 20: 593 – 8

[Writer's cramp treated with botulinum injections]. Koelman JH et al. Ned Tijdschr Geneeskd. 1998; 142: 1768 – 71

2.4.2 Lower Extremities

Botulinum toxin therapy for limb dystonias. Yoshimura DM et al. Neurology 1992; 42: 627 – 30

The use of botulinum toxin to treat "striatal" toes [letter]. Giladi N et al. J Neurol Neurosurg Psychiatry 1994; 57: 659

Dystonic posture of lower extremities associated with myelomeningocele: successful treatment with botulinum A toxin in a six-month-old child. Heinen F et al. Neuropediatrics 1995; 26: 214 – 6

Treatment of nonoccupational limb and trunk dystonia with botulinum toxin. Quirk JA et al. Mov Disord. 1996; 11: 377 – 83

2.5 Axial Dystonia

Treatment of nonoccupational limb and trunk dystonia with botulinum toxin. Quirk JA et al. Mov Disord. 1996; 11: 377 – 83

Extensor truncal dystonia: successful treatment with botulinum toxin injections. Comella CL et al. J Mov Disord. 1998; 13: 552 – 5

3 Spastic Conditions

Botulinum toxin in treating spasticity. Das TK, Park DM. Br J Clin Pract. 1989; 43: 401 – 3

Effect of treatment with botulinum toxin on spasticity. Das TK, Park DM. Postgrad Med J. 1989; 65: 208 – 10

Treatment of spasticity with botulinum toxin: a double-blind study. Snow BJ et al. Ann Neurol. 1990; 28: 512 – 5

Treatment of spasticity with botulinum toxin [letter]. Borodic GE et al. Ann Neurol. 1992; 31: 113

Local botulinum toxin in the treatment of spastic drop foot. Dengler R et al. J Neurol. 1992; 239: 375 – 8

Botulinum toxin for the treatment of spasticity in multiple sclerosis. New observations. Borg-Stein J et al. Am J Phys Med Rehabil. 1993; 72: 364 – 8

Local treatment of dystonia and spasticity with injections of botulinum-A toxin. Calne S. Axone 1993; 14: 85 – 8

Botulinum toxin treatment for lower limb extensor spasticity in chronic hemiparetic patients. Hesse S et al. J Neurol Neurosurg Psychiatry 1994; 57: 1321 – 4

Treatment of chronic limb spasticity with botulinum toxin A [see comments]. Comment in: J Neurol Neurosurg Psychiatry 1995; 59: 562; Dunne JW et al. J Neurol Neurosurg Psychiatry 1995; 58: 232 – 5

Botulinum toxin A for spasticity, muscle spasms, and rigidity. Grazko MA et al. Neurology 1995; 45: 712 – 7

Use of botulinum toxin in stroke patients with severe upper limb spasticity. Bhakta BB et al. J Neurol Neurosurg Psychiatry 1996; 61: 30 – 5

A randomised, double blind, placebo controlled trial of botulinum toxin in the treatment of spastic foot in hemiparetic patients. Burbaud P et al. J Neurol Neurosurg Psychiatry 1996; 61: 265 – 9

Comparison of two injection techniques using botulinum toxin in spastic hemiplegia. Childers MK et al. Am J Phys Med Rehabil. 1996; 75: 462 – 9

The effect of botulinum toxin A on the function if a person with poststroke quadriplegia. Cromwell SJ, Paquette VL. Phys Ther. 1996; 76: 395 – 402

[Botulinum toxin therapy in rehabilitation neurology]. Dressler D et al. Nervenarzt 1996; 67: 686 – 94

Ankle muscle activity before and after botulinum toxin therapy for lower limb extensor spasticity in chronic hemiparetic patients. Hesse S et al. Stroke 1996; 27: 455 – 60

Spasticity after stroke. Epidemiology and optimal treatment. O'Brien CF et al. Drugs Aging 1996; 9: 332 – 40

Botulinum toxin A in the treatment of spasticity: functional implications and patient selection. Pierson SH et al. Arch Phys Med Rehabil. 1996; 77: 717 – 21

Botulinum toxin type A in the treatment of upper extremity spasticity: a randomized, double-blind, placebo-controlled trial. Simpson DM et al. Neurology 1996; 46: 1306 – 10

Botulinum toxin in severe upper extremity spasticity among patients with traumatic brain injury: an open-labeled trial. Yablon SA et al. Neurology 1996; 47: 939 – 44

Management of spasticity. Hesse S, Mauritz KH. Curr Opin Neurol. 1997; 10: 498 – 501

Botulinum toxin type A for the treatment of arm and hand spasticity in stroke patients. Sampaio C et al. Clin Rehabil. 1997; 11: 3 – 7

Botulinum toxin type A and short-term electrical stimulation in the treatment of upper limb flexor spasticity after stroke: a randomized, double-blind, placebo-controlled trial. Hesse S et al. Clin Rehabil. 1998; 12: 381 – 8

A study of the effectiveness of botulinum toxin type A (Dysport) in the management of muscle spasticity. Watanabe Y et al. Disabil Rehabil. 1998; 20: 62 – 5

Botulinum toxin A in hamstring spasticity. Corry IS et al. Gait Posture 1999; 10: 206 – 10

4   Cerebral Palsy

Botulinum toxin in the management of the lower limb in cerebral palsy. Cosgrove AP et al. Dev Med Child Neurol. 1994; 36: 386 – 96

Management of spasticity in cerebral palsy with botulinum-A toxin: report of a preliminary, randomized, double-blind trial. Koman LA et al. J Pediatr Orthop. 1994; 14: 299 – 303

Botulinum toxin in the treatment of cerebral palsy. Denislic M, Meh D. Neuropediatrics 1995; 26: 249 – 52

Botulinum toxin for spasticity and athetosis in children with cerebral palsy. Gooch JL, Sandell TV. Arch Phys Med Rehabil. 1996; 77: 508 – 11

Dosing, administration, and a treatment algorithm for use of botulinum toxin A for adult-onset spasticity. Spasticity Study Group. Brin MF. Muscle Nerve Suppl. 1997; 6: S208 – 20

Treatment of cerebral palsy with botulinum toxin A: functional benefit and reduction of disability. Three case reports. Mall V et al. Pediatr Rehabil. 1997; 1: 235 – 7

Cerebral palsy: a rational approach to a treatment protocol, and the role of botulinum toxin in treatment. Russman BS et al. Muscle Nerve Suppl. 1997; 6: S181 – 93

Clinical trials of botulinum toxin in the treatment of spasticity. Simpson DM. Muscle Nerve Suppl. 1997; 6: S169 – 75

The role of botulinum toxin in the treatment of lower limb spasticity in children with cerebral palsy–a pilot study. Zelnik N et al. Isr J Med Sci. 1997; 33: 129 – 33

Use of botulinum toxin injection in 17 children with spastic cerebral palsy. Wong V. Pediatr Neurol. 1998; 18: 124 – 31

Position paper on the use of botulinum toxin in cerebral palsy. UK Botulinum Toxin and Cerebral Palsy Working Party. Carr LJ et al. Arch Dis Child 1998; 79: 271 – 3

Management of spasticity in children: part 1: chemical denervation. Gormley ME Jr. J Head Trauma Rehabil. 1999; 14: 97 – 9

Botulinum toxin A in the management of spastic gait disorders in children and young adults with cerebral palsy: a randomized, double-blind study of "high-dose" versus "low-dose" treatment. Wissel J et al. Gait Posture 1999; 10: 1 – 9

Double-blind study of botulinum A toxin injections into the gastrocnemius muscle in patients with cerebral palsy. Sutherland DH et al. Gait Posture 1999; 10: 1 – 9

5   Hemifacial Spasm

Blepharospasm, Meige syndrome, and hemifacial spasm: treatment with botulinum toxin. Mauriello JA Jr. Neurology 1985; 35: 1499 – 500

Treatment of facial spasm with oculinum (Clostridium botulinum toxin): a preliminary report. Biglan AW et al. Am J Otol. 1986; 7: 65 – 70

Treatment of facial spasm with Oculinum (C. botulinum toxin). Biglan AW, May M. J Pediatr Ophthalmol Strabismus 1986; 23: 216 – 21

Botulinum toxin treatment of hemifacial spasm. Elston JS. J Neurol Neurosurg Psychiatry 1986; 49: 827 – 9

Treatment of facial spasm with botulinum toxin. An interim report. Frueh BR, Musch DC. Ophthalmology 1986; 93: 917 – 23

Botulinum toxin for benign essential blepharospasm, hemifacial spasm and age-related lower eyelid entropion. Carruthers J, Stubbs HA. Can J Neurol Sci. 1987; 14: 42 – 5

Use of botulinum toxin in the treatment of one hundred patients with facial dyskinesias. Mauriello JA Jr et al. Ophthalmology 1987; 94: 976 – 9

Use of botulinum toxin in blepharospasm and other facial spasms. Ruusuvaara P, Setala K. Acta Ophthalmol Copenh. 1987; 65: 313 – 9

Management of facial spasm with Clostridium botulinum toxin, type A. Biglan AW et al. Arch Otolaryngol Head Neck Surg. 1988; 114: 1407 – 12

Localized injections of botulinum toxin for the treatment of focal dystonia and hemifacial spasm. Brin MF et al. Adv Neurol. 1988; 50: 599 – 608

Botulinum toxin injections in the treatment of blepharospasm, hemifacial spasm, and eyelid fasciculations. Kraft SP, Lang AE. Can J Neurol Sci. 1988; 15: 276 – 80

Cranial dystonia, blepharospasm and hemifacial spasm: clinical features and treatment, including the use of botulinum toxin. Kraft SP, Lang AE. Can Med Assoc J. 1988; 139: 837 – 44

Botulinum toxin injection therapy for hemifacial spasm. Tolosa E et al. Adv Neurol. 1988; 49: 479 – 91

Botulinum toxin therapy in hemifacial spasm: clinical and electrophysiologic studies. Geller BD. Muscle Nerve 1989; 12: 716 – 22

Botulinum toxin in the treatment of hemifacial spasm. Chong-PN. Singapore Med J. 1990; 469 – 71

Botulinum A toxin treatment for eyelid spasm, spasmodic torticollis and apraxia of eyelid opening. Defazio G et al. Ital J Neurol Sci. 1990; 11: 275 – 80

Eyelid movements before and after botulinum therapy in patients with lid spasm. Manning KA et al. Ann Neurol. 1990; 28: 653 – 60

Long-term treatment of involuntary facial spasms using botulinum toxin. Ruusuvaara P, Setala K. Acta Ophthalmol Copenh. 1990; 68: 331 – 8

Botulinum toxin in the treatment of facial dyskinesias. Chong PN et al. Ann Acad Med Singapore 1991; 20: 223 – 7

Natural history of treatment of facial dyskinesias with botulinum toxin: a study of 50 consecutive patients over seven years. Mauriello JA, Aljian J. Br J Ophthalmol. 1991; 75: 737 – 9

Treatment of blepharospasm and hemifacial spasm with botulinum A toxin: a Canadian multicentre study. Taylor JD et al. Can J Ophthalmol. 1991; 26: 133 – 8

Botulinum toxin injections for treatment of blepharospasm and hemifacial spasm. Wirtschafter JD, Rubenfeld M. Int Ophthalmol Clin. 1991; 31: 117 – 32

Contralateral injections of botulinum A toxin for the treatment of hemifacial spasm to achieve increased facial symmetry [see comments]. Borodic GE et al. Plast Reconstr Surg. 1992; 90: 972 – 7; discussion 978 – 9

The management of blepharospasm and hemifacial spasm. Elston JS. J Neurol. 1992; 239: 5 – 8

Two hundred and fifty patients with hemifacial spasm treated with botulinum toxin injection. Poungvarin N, Viriyavejakul A. J Med Assoc Thai. 1992; 75: 199–203

Treatment of hemifacial spasm with botulinum toxin. Yoshimura DM et al. Muscle Nerve 1992; 15: 1045–9

Botulinum toxin treatment in patients with focal dystonia and hemifacial spasm. A multicenter study of the Italian Movement Disorder Group. Berardelli A et al. Ital J Neurol Sci. 1993; 14: 361–7

Botulinum a toxin treatment of hemifacial spasm and blepharospasm. Park YC et al. J Korean Med Sci. 1993; 8: 334–40

A comparative study of tear secretion in blepharospasm and hemifacial spasm patients treated with botulinum toxin. Price J, O'Day J. J Clin Neuroophthalmol. 1993; 13: 67–71

The use of botulinum toxin type A for the treatment of facial spasm. Serrano LA. Bol Asoc Med P R. 1993; 85: 7–11

Botulinum toxin treatment in patients with hemifacial spasm. Laskawi R. Eur Arch Otorhinolaryngol. 1994; 251: 271–4

Efficacy and side effects of botulinum toxin treatment for blepharospasm and hemifacial spasm. Price J, O'Day J. Aust NZ J Ophthalmol. 1994; 22: 255–60

Chemomyectomy of the orbicularis oculi muscles for the treatment of localized hemifacial spasm. Wirtschafter JD. J Neuroophthalmol. 1994; 14: 199–204

Treatment of hemifacial spasm with botulinum toxin. Value of preinjection electromyography abnormalities for predicting postinjection lower facial paresis. Angibaud G et al. Eur Neurol. 1995; 35: 43–5

Botulinum toxin-A for the treatment of hemifacial spasm. Cuevas C et al. Arch Med Res. 1995; 26: 405–8

Botulinum toxin A injection in the treatment of hemifacial spasm. Chen RS et al. Acta Neurol Scand. 1996; 94: 207–11

Treatment choices of 119 patients with hemifacial spasm over 11 years. Mauriello JA Jr et al. Clin Neurol Neurosurg. 1996; 98: 213–6

Long term results of botulinum toxin type A (Dysport) in the treatment of hemifacial spasm: a report of 175 cases. Jitpimolmard S et al. J Neurol Neurosurg Psychiatry 1998; 64: 751–7

6   Facial Synkinesias

Management of facial spasm with Clostridium botulinum toxin, type A (Oculinum) [see comments]. Biglan AW et al. Arch Otolaryngol Head Neck Surg. 1988; 114: 1407–12

Bell's palsy: management of sequelae using EMG rehabilitation, botulinum toxin, and surgery. May M et al. Am J Otol. 1989; 10: 220–9

Botulinum toxin to suppress hyperkinesias after hypoglossal-facial nerve anastomosis. Dressler D, Schonle PW. Eur Arch Otorhinolaryngol. 1990; 247: 391–2

Botulinum toxin injections in the treatment of seventh nerve misdirection. Putterman AM. Am J Ophthalmol. 1990; 110: 205–6

Management of facial synkinesis with Clostridium botulinum toxin injection. Mountain RE et al. Clin Otolaryngol. 1992; 17: 223 – 4

Orbicular synkinesis after facial paralysis: treatment with botulinum toxin. Roggenkamper P et al. Doc Ophthalmol. 1994; 86: 395 – 402

Treatment of facial synkinesis and facial asymmetry with botulinum toxin type A following facial nerve palsy. Armstrong MW et al. Clin Otolaryngol. 1996; 21: 15 – 20

Combination of hypoglossal-facial nerve anastomosis and botulinum-toxin injections to optimize mimic rehabilitation after removal of acoustic neurinomas. Laskawi R. Plast Reconstr Surg. 1997; 99: 1006 – 11

7   Facial Asymmetries

Botulinum toxin: a treatment for facial asymmetry caused by facial nerve paralysis. Clark RP, Berris CE. Plast Reconstr Surg. 1989; 84: 353 – 5

Botulinum A toxin injection in patients with facial nerve palsy. Smet Dieleman H et al. Acta Otorhinolaryngol Belg. 1993; 47: 359 – 63

Treatment of facial synkinesis and facial asymmetry with botulinum toxin type A following facial nerve palsy. Armstrong MW et al. Clin Otolaryngol. 1996; 21: 15 – 20

8   Hyperactive Facial Lines

Botulinum toxin for the treatment of hyperfunctional lines of the face [see comments]. Blitzer A et al. Arch Otolaryngol Head Neck Surg. 1993; 119: 1018 – 22

Botulinum toxin A for hyperkinetic facial lines: results of a double-blind, placebo-controlled study. Keen M et al. Plast Reconstr Surg. 1994; 94: 94 – 9

Botulinum A exotoxin use in clinical dermatology. Carruthers A et al. J Am Acad Dermatol. 1996; 34: 788 – 97

The use of botulinum A toxin to ameliorate facial kinetic frown lines. Foster JA et al. Ophthalmology 1996; 103: 618 – 22

Cosmetic denervation of the muscles of facial expression with botulinum toxin. A dose-response study. Garcia A, Fulton JE Jr. Dermatol Surg. 1996; 22: 39 – 43

Review of the use of botulinum toxin for aesthetic improvement. Garner W. Ann Plast Surg. 1996; 36: 192

Botulinum toxin type A injection for hyperfunctional facial lines [letter]. Herwig SR. Laryngoscope 1996; 106: 1187

Botulinum A exotoxin for glabellar folds: a double-blind, placebo-controlled study with an electromyographic injection technique. Lowe NJ et al. J Am Acad Dermatol. 1996; 35: 569 – 72

The management of hyperfunctional facial lines with botulinum toxin. A collaborative study of 210 injection sites in 162 patients. Blitzer A et al. J Otolaryngol. 1997; 26: 92 – 6

Cosmetic uses of botulinum A exotoxin. Carruthers A, Carruthers J. Adv Dermatol. 1997; 12: 325 – 47; discussion 348

Cosmetic uses of botulinum A exotoxin. Carruthers A, Carruthers J. Dermatol Nurs. 1997; 9: 329 – 33, 365

Cosmetic botulinum toxin injections. Carter SR, Seiff SR. Arch Otolaryngol Head Neck Surg. 1997; 123: 389 – 92

Cosmetic upper-facial rejuvenation with botulinum. Ellis DA, Tan AK. Arch Otolaryngol Head Neck Surg. 1997; 123: 321 – 6

Chemical browlift. Frankel AS, Kamer FM. Ann Plast Surg. 1997; 39: 447 – 53

Local injection into mimetic muscles of botulinum toxin A for the treatment of facial lines. Guerrissi J, Sarkissian P. Int Ophthalmol Clin. 1997; 37: 69 – 79

Patient selection in the treatment of glabellar wrinkles with botulinum toxin type A injection. Pribitkin EA et al. Arch Otolaryngol Head Neck Surg. 1997; 123: 321 – 6

Patient selection in the treatment of glabellar wrinkles with botulinum toxin type A injection. Pribitkin EA et al. Adv Dermatol. 1997; 12: 325 – 47; discussion 348

Treatment of hyperfunctional lines of the face with botulinum toxin A. Binder WJ et al. Dermatol Surg. 1998; 24: 1189 – 94

Cosmetic use of botulinum A exotoxin for the aging neck. Brandt FS, Bellman B. Dermatol Surg. 1998; 24: 1216 – 8

Clinical indications and injection technique for the cosmetic use of botulinum A exotoxin. Carruthers A, Carruthers J. Dermatol Surg. 1998; 24: 1181 – 3

Oculoplastic experience with the cosmetic use of botulinum A exotoxin. Edelstein C et al. Dermatol Surg. 1998; 24: 1198 – 205

Cosmetic indications for botulinum A toxin. Foster JA et al. Dermatol Surg. 1998; 24: 1249 – 54

Botulinum toxin for the correction of hyperkinetic facial lines. Goodman G. Australas J Dermatol 1998; 39: 158 – 63

Botulinum A toxin for glabellar wrinkles. Dose and response. Hankins CL et al. Arch Otolaryngol Head Neck Surg. 1998; 124: 321 – 3

[Botulinum toxin and facial wrinkles: a new injection procedure]. Le Louarn C. Ann Chir Plast Esthet. 1998; 43: 526 – 33

[Botulinum toxin and facial wrinkles: a new injection procedure]. Le Louarn C. Aesthetic Plast Surg. 1998; 22: 366 – 71

Botulinum toxin type A for facial rejuvenation. United States and United Kingdom perspectives. Lowe NJ. Dermatol Surg. 1998; 24: 1208 – 12

Eyebrow asymmetry: ways of correction. Muhlbauer W, Holm C. Ann Pharmacother. 1998; 32: 1365 – 7

Aesthetic uses of botulinum toxin A. Niamtu J 3rd. Dermatol Surg. 1998; 24: 1232 – 4

Botulinum toxin type A injection for the treatment of frown lines. Song KH. Semin Ophthalmol. 1998; 13: 142 – 8

The cosmetic uses of Botulinum toxin type A. Benedetto AV. J Oral Maxillofac Surg. 1999; 57: 1228 – 33

Facial rejuvenation with botulinum. Ellis DA et al. Plast Reconstr Surg 1999; 103: 701 – 13

Botox for the treatment of dynamic and hyperkinetic facial lines and furrows: adjunctive use in facial aesthetic surgery. Fagien S. Plast Reconstr Surg. 1999; 103:

656–63; discussion 664–5 Published erratum appears in Plast Reconstr Surg 1999; 103(3) following table of contents

Nonsurgical treatment of platysmal bands with injection of botulinum toxin A. Kane MA. Plast Reconstr Surg. 1999; 103: 645–52; discussion 653–5

Periorbital rejuvenation: a review of dermatologic treatments. Manaloto RM, Alster TS. Dermatol Surg. 1999; 25: 1–9

Botulinum A exotoxin for the management of platysma bands. Matarasso A. Plast Reconstr Surg. 1999; 103: 645–53

Complications of botulinum A exotoxin for hyperfunctional lines. Matarasso SL. Int J Dermatol. 1999; 38: 641–55

9 Ocular Misalignment

9.1 Mixed Strabismus

Botulinum toxin injection into extraocular muscles as an alternative to strabismus surgery. Scott AB. J Pediatr Ophthalmol Strabismus. 1980; 17: 21–5

Botulinum toxin injection into extraocular muscles as an alternative to strabismus surgery. Scott AB. Ophthalmology 1980; 87: 1044–9

Botulinum toxin injection of eye muscles to correct strabismus. Scott AB. Trans Am Ophthalmol Soc. 1981; 79: 734–70

The use of botulinum toxin A in the treatment of strabismus. Elston JS. Trans Ophthalmol Soc UK. 1985; 104: 208–10

Use of botulinum toxin for treatment of strabismus, a preliminary report. Walden PG, Biglan AW. Trans Pa Acad Ophthalmol Otolaryngol. 1985; 37: 136–42

Ptosis associated with botulinum toxin treatment of strabismus and blepharospasm. Burns CL et al. Ophthalmology 1986; 93: 1621–7

Botulinum toxin therapy for strabismus and blepharospasm: Bascom Palmer Eye Institute experience. Flynn JT, Bachynski B. Trans New Orleans Acad Ophthalmol. 1986; 34: 73–88

Botulinum toxin injections in strabismus. Jampolsky A. Trans New Orleans Acad Ophthalmol. 1986; 34: 526–36

Injection of type A botulinum toxin into extraocular muscles for correction of strabismus. Flanders M et al. Can J Ophthalmol. 1987; 22: 212–7

Botulinum vs adjustable suture surgery in the treatment of horizontal misalignment in adult patients lacking fusion. Carruthers JD et al. Arch Ophthalmol. 1990; 108: 1432–5

Botulinum toxin for the treatment of blepharospasm and strabismus. Paul TO. West J Med. 1990; 153: 187

When considering Oculinum (botulinum toxin type A) injection for the treatment of strabismus, can the surgeon anticipate different results in patients who have had previous strabismus surgery? Scott AB. Arch Ophthalmol. 1991; 109: 1510

9.2 Paralytic Strabismus

Paralytic strabismus: the role of botulinum toxin. Elston JS, Lee JP. Br J Ophthalmol. 1985; 69: 891–6

Botulinum toxin injection in the management of lateral rectus paresis. Scott AB, Kraft SP. Ophthalmology 1985; 92: 676–83

Treatment of sixth nerve palsy in adults with combined botulinum toxin chemodenervation and surgery. Fitzsimons R et al. Ophthalmology 1988; 95: 1535 – 42

The role of botulinum toxin in the management of sixth nerve palsy. Fitzsimons R et al. Eye 1989; 3: 391 – 400

Vertical rectus muscle transposition and botulinum toxin (Oculinum) to medial rectus for abducens palsy [see comments]. Rosenbaum AL et al. Arch Ophthalmol. 1989; 107: 820 – 3

Early and late botulinum toxin treatment of acute sixth nerve palsy. Murray AD. Aust NZ J Ophthalmol. 1989; 17: 239 – 45

Long-term results: botulinum for sixth nerve palsy. Wagner RS, Frohman LP. J Pediatr Ophthalmol Strabismus 1989; 26: 106 – 8

Vertical rectus muscle transposition with intraoperative botulinum injection for treatment of chronic sixth nerve palsy. McManaway JW 3 d et al. Graefes Arch Clin Exp Ophthalmol. 1990; 228: 401 – 6

Modern management of sixth nerve palsy. Lee J. Am J Ophthalmol. 1991; 112: 381 – 4

Treatment of unilateral acute sixth-nerve palsy with botulinum toxin. Metz HS, Dickey CF. Am J Ophthalmol 1991; 112: 381 – 4

Early botulinum toxin treatment of acute sixth nerve palsy. Murray AD. Eye 1991; 5: 45 – 7

The role of botulinum toxin in third nerve palsy. Saad N, Lee J. Aust NZ J Ophthalmol. 1992; 20: 41 – 6

Botulinum toxin in the treatment of paralytic strabismus and essential blepharospasm. Thomas R et al. Indian J Ophthalmol. 1993; 41 : 121 – 4

Results of a prospective randomized trial of botulinum toxin therapy in acute unilateral sixth nerve palsy. Lee J et al. J Pediatr Ophthalmol Strabismus 1994; 31: 283 – 6

9.3 Concomitant Strabismus

Treatment of strabismus in adults with botulinum toxin A. Elston JS et al. Br J Ophthalmol. 1985; 69: 718 – 24

Factors influencing success and dose-effect relation of botulinum A treatment. Abbasoglu OE et al. Eye 1996; 10: 385 – 91

9.4 Strabismus after Retinal Detachment Surgery

Botulinum treatment of strabismus following retinal detachment surgery. Scott AB. Arch Ophthalmol. 1990; 108: 509 – 10

Use of botulinum toxin in strabismus after retinal detachment surgery. Petitto VB, Buckley EG. Ophthalmology 1991; 98: 509 – 12; discussion 512 – 3

9.5 Strabismus after Cataract Surgery

Persistent binocular diplopia after cataract surgery. Hamed LM et al. Am J Ophthalmol. 1987; 103: 741 – 4

9.6　Strabismus after Aphakia

Binocular diplopia in unilateral aphakia: the role of botulinum toxin. Hakin KN, Lee JP. Eye 1991; 5: 447 – 50

9.7　Myositic Strabismus

Management of strabismus due to orbital myositis. Bessant DA, Lee JP. Eye 1995; 9: 558 – 63

9.8　Myopathic Strabismus

Injection treatment of endocrine orbital myopathy. Scott AB. Doc Ophthalmol. 1984; 58: 141 – 5

Botulinum toxin for the treatment of dysthyroid ocular myopathy. Dunn WJ et al. Ophthalmology 1986; 93: 470 – 5

Botulinum toxin therapy in dysthyroid strabismus. Lyons CJ et al. Eye 1990; 4: 538 – 42

What is the role of botulinum toxin in the treatment of dysthyroid strabismus? Gair EJ et al. J AAPOS 1999; 3: 272 – 4

9.9　Dissociated Vertical Deviation

Botulinum toxin injection into the superior rectus muscle of the non-dominant eye for dissociated vertical deviation. McNeer KW. J Pediatr Ophthalmol Strabismus 1989; 26: 162 – 4

9.10　Botulinum Toxin Therapy as Adjunct to Strabismus Surgery

An investigation of the clinical use of botulinum toxin A as a postoperative adjustment procedure in the therapy of strabismus. McNeer KW. J Pediatr Ophthalmol Strabismus 1990; 27: 3 – 9

9.11　Esotropia

Botulinum alignment for congenital esotropia [see comments]. Ing MR. Ophthalmology 1993; 100: 318 – 22

Observations on bilateral simultaneous botulinum toxin injection in infantile esotropia. McNeer KW et al. J Pediatr Ophthalmol Strabismus 1994; 31: 214 – 9.

9.12　Exotropia

[Surgical and botulinum toxin treatment in two cases of abnormal retinal correspondence-exotropia with congenital homonymous hemianopsia]. Iwashige H et al. Nippon Ganka Gakkai Zasshi 1995; 99: 1036 – 44

[The dose-response relationship in treatment of strabismus with botulinum toxin] Kimura H et al. Nippon Ganka Gakkai Zasshi 1996; 100: 213 – 8

Long-term results of botulinum toxin in consecutive and secondary exotropia: outcome in patients initially treated with botulinum toxin. Lawson JM et al. J AAPOS 1998; 2 : 195 – 200

10   Achalasia

Botulinum toxin for achalasia [letter]. Pasricha PJ et al. Lancet 1993; 341: 244 – 5
Treatment of achalasia with intrasphincteric injection of botulinum toxin. A pilot trial. Pasricha PJ et al. Ann Intern Med. 1994; 121: 590 – 1
Use of botulin A toxin in achalasia. al-Karawi MA et al. Endoscopy 1995; 27: 217
Treatment of achalasia in Chagas' disease with botulinum toxin [letter]. Ferrari AP Jr et al. N Engl J Med. 1995; 332: 824 – 5
Achalasia. A new modality for treatment. Mitchell RE Jr et al. Va Med Q. 1995; 122: 184 – 5
Intrasphincteric botulinum toxin for the treatment of achalasia [see comments]; [published erratum appears in N Engl J Med. 1995; 333: 75]; Comment in: N Engl J Med. 1995; 332: 815 – 6; Comment in: ACP J Club 1995; 123: 38. Pasricha PJ et al. N Engl J Med. 1995; 332: 774 – 8
Endoscopic intrasphincteric injection of botulinum toxin for the treatment of achalasia. Rollan A et al. J Clin Gastroenterol. 1995; 20: 189 – 91
Controlled trial of botulinum toxin injection versus placebo and pneumatic dilation in achalasia. Annese V et al. Gastroenterology 1996; 111: 1418 – 24
Perendoscopic injection of botulinum toxin is effective in achalasia after failure of myotomy or pneumatic dilation. Annese V et al. Gastrointest Endosc. 1996; 44: 461 – 5
Long-term outcome of botulinum toxin in the treatment of achalasia [letter]. Birgisson S, Richter JE. Gastroenterology 1996; 111: 1162 – 3
Symptomatic improvement in achalasia after botulinum toxin injection of the lower esophageal sphincter. Fishman VM et al. Am J Gastroenterol. 1996; 91: 1724 – 30
Botulinum toxin in hypertensive lower esophageal sphincter [letter]. Jones MP. Am J Gastroenterol. 1996; 91: 1283 – 4
Use of high-resolution endoscopic ultrasonography to assess esophageal wall damage after pneumatic dilation and botulinum toxin injection to treat achalasia. Schiano TD et al. Gastrointest Endosc. 1996; 44: 151 – 7
Role of botulinum toxin in treatment of achalasia cardia [see comments]; Comment in: Indian J Gastroenterol. 1996; 15: 82 – 5. Sood A et al. Indian J Gastroenterol. 1996; 15: 97 – 8
Use of botulinum toxin for diagnosis and management of cricopharyngeal achalasia. Blitzer A, Brin MF. Otolaryngol Head Neck Surg. 1997; 116: 328 – 30
Recent advances in the treatment of achalasia. Pasricha PJ, Kalloo AN. Gastrointest Endosc Clin N Am. 1997; 7: 191 – 206
Botulinum toxin A for the treatment of achalasia. Rodriguez Cruz E et al. Bol Asoc Med P R. 1997; 89: 57 – 9
Botulinum toxin in long-term therapy for achalasia. Annese V et al. Ann Intern Med. 1998; 128: 696
Intrasphincteric injection of botulinum toxin is effective in long-term treatment of esophageal achalasia. Annese V et al. Muscle Nerve 1998; 21: 1540 – 2
[Achalasia: botulinus toxin, interventional balloon dilatation, myotomy] Schneider JH et al. Schweiz Rundsch Med Prax. 1998; 87: 1213 – 21

Botox injection for achalasia: a modified technique. Goldstein JA, Barkin JS. Gastrointest Endosc 1999; 49: 272 – 3

Early experience with intrasphincteric botulinum toxin in the treatment of achalasia. Greaves RR et al. Endoscopy 1999; 31: 352 – 8; Aliment Pharmacol Ther. 1999; 13: 1221 – 5

Esophageal achalasia: intrasphincteric injection of botulinum toxin A versus balloon dilation. Muehldorfer SM et al. Endoscopy 1999; 31: 517 – 21

Long-term efficacy of Botulinum toxin in classical achalasia: a prospective study. Kolbasnik J et al. Am J Gastroenterol. 1999; 94: 3434 – 9

Botulinum toxin versus pneumatic dilatation in the treatment of achalasia: a randomised trial. Vaezi MF et al. Gut 1999; 44: 231 – 9

Long-term results of endoscopic injection of botulinum toxin in elderly achalasic patients with tortuous megaesophagus or epiphrenic diverticulum. Wehrmann T et al. Gastrointest Endosc. 1999; 49: 272 – 3

Video-assisted surgical management of achalasia of the esophagus. Wiechmann RJ et al. J Thorac Cardiovasc Surg. 1999; 118: 916 – 23

11   Anal Fissures

Use of botulinum toxin in anal fissure [letter]. Jost WH, Schimrigk K. Dis Colon Rectum 1993; 36: 974

Botulinum toxin for chronic anal fissure [see comments]. Gui D et al. Lancet 1994; 344: 1127 – 8

Botulinum toxin in the management of anal fissure: innovative use of a familiar agent. Goel AK, Seenu V. Trop Gastroenterol. 1995; 16: 68 – 9

Perianal thrombosis following injection therapy into the external anal sphincter using botulin toxin [letter]. Jost WH et al. Dis Colon Rectum 1995; 38: 781

Botulinum toxin in therapy of anal fissure [letter; comment]. Jost WH, Schimrigk K. Lancet 1995; 345: 188 – 9

Anorectal disorders. Janicke DM, Pundt MR. Emerg Med Clin North Am. 1996; 14: 757 – 88

Aetiology and treatment of anal fissure. Lund JN, Scholefield JH. Br J Surg. 1996; 83: 1335 – 44

The management of chronic fissure in-ano with botulinum toxin. Mason PF et al. J R Coll Surg Edinb. 1996; 41: 235 – 8

Patient selection and treatment modalities for chronic anal fissure. Sharp FR. Am J Surg. 1996; 171: 512 – 5

One hundred cases of anal fissure treated with botulin toxin: early and long-term results. Jost WH. Dis Colon Rectum 1997; 40: 1029 – 32

The management of chronic fissure in ano with botulinum toxin. Moore AP. J R Coll Surg Edinb. 1997; 42: 289

The use of botulinum toxin for anal fissure. Parikh VA. J R Coll Surg Edinb. 1997; 42: 288 – 9.

The management of chronic fissure in ano with botulinum toxin. Wannas HR. J R Coll Surg Edinb. 1997; 42: 289 – 90

A comparison of botulinum toxin and saline for the treatment of chronic anal fissure. Maria G et al. N Engl J Med. 1998; 338: 217–20

Botulinum toxin injections in the internal anal sphincter for the treatment of chronic anal fissure: long-term results after two different dosage regimens. Maria G et al. Ann Surg 1998; 228: 664–9

Treatment of chronic anal fissure. Perez-Miranda M, Jimenez JM. N Engl J Med 1998; 338: 1698–9

Botulinum toxin promoted healing and relieved symptoms of chronic anal fissure. Phillips RKS. Gut 1998; 43: 601

A comparison of injections of botulinum toxin and topical nitroglycerin ointment for the treatment of chronic anal fissure. Brisinda G et al. N Engl J Med. 1999; 341: 65–9

The expanding spectrum of clinical uses for botulinum toxin: healing of chronic anal fissures. Hasler WL. Gastroenterology 1999; 116: 221–3

Repeat botulin toxin injections in anal fissure: in patients with relapse and after insufficient effect of first treatment. Jost WH, Schrank B. Dig Dis Sci. 1999; 44: 1588–9

Nonsurgical treatment modalities for chronic anal fissure using botulinum toxin. Madalinski MH. Gastroenterology 1999; 117: 516–7

Therapeutic effects of different doses of botulinum toxin in chronic anal fissure. Minguez M et al. Dis Colon Rectum 1999; 42: 1016–21

12 Exocrine Gland Hyperactivity

12.1 Frey Syndrome

Frey's syndrome: treatment with botulinum toxin. Drobik C, Laskawi R. Acta Otolaryngol Stockh. 1995; 115: 459–61

Botulinum toxin in the therapy of gustatory sweating. Schulze Bonhage A et al. J Neurol. 1996; 243: 143–6

Frey's syndrome: treatment with botulinum toxin. Bjerkhoel A, Trobbe O. J Laryngol Otol. 1997; 111: 839–44

Treatment of gustatory sweating with botulinum toxin. Naumann M et al. Ann Neurol. 1997; 42: 973–5

[Treatment of Frey's syndrome with botulinum A toxin]. Braunius WW, Gerrits MA. Ned Tijdschr Geneeskd. 1998; 142: 859–63

Botulinum toxin type A for Frey's syndrome: a preliminary prospective study. Laccourreye O et al. Ann Otol Rhinol Laryngol. 1998; 107: 52–5

Up-to-date report of botulinum toxin type A treatment in patients with gustatory sweating (Frey's syndrome). Laskawi R et al. Laryngoscope 1998; 108: 381–4

Botulinum toxoid in the management of gustatory sweating (Frey's syndrome) after superficial parotidectomy. Birch JF et al. Br J Plast Surg. 1999; 52: 230–1

Recurrent gustatory sweating (Frey syndrome) after intracutaneous injection of botulinum toxin type A: incidence, management, and outcome. Laccourreye O et al. Arch Otolaryngol Head Neck Surg. 1999; 125: 283–6

[Severe Frey syndrome after parotidectomy: treatment with botulinum neurotoxin type A]. Laccourreye O et al. Ann Otolaryngol Chir Cervicofac. 1999; 116: 137–42

12.2 Crocodile Tears Syndrome

Successful treatment of crocodile tears by injection of botulinum toxin into the lacrimal gland: a case report. Riemann R et al. Br J Plast Surg. 1999; 52: 230–1

12.3 Hyperhidrosis

Botulinum toxin and sweating [letter]. Bushara KO, Park DM. J Neurol Neurosurg Psychiatry 1994; 57: 1437–8

Botulinum toxin–a possible new treatment for axillary hyperhidrosis. Bushara KO et al. Clin Exp Dermatol. 1996; 21: 276–8

Botulinum A toxin injection in focal hyperhidrosis [letter]. Schnider P et al. Br J Dermatol. 1996; 134: 1160–1

Botulinum toxin for palmar hyperhidrosis [letter]. Naumann M et al. Lancet 1997; 349: 252

Double-blind trial of botulinum A toxin for the treatment of focal hyperhidrosis of the palms. Schnider P et al. Br J Dermatol. 1997; 136: 548–52

[New therapeutic principle in severe hyperhidrosis. Botulinum toxin injections can replace cutting of nerves]. Aquilonius SM, Naver H. Lakartidningen 1998; 95: 3658–9

Botulinum A neurotoxin for axillary hyperhidrosis. No sweat Botox. Glogau RG. Dermatol Surg. 1998; 24: 817–9

Follow-up of patients with axillary hyperhidrosis after botulinum toxin injection. Heckmann M et al. Arch Dermatol. 1998; 134: 1298–9

Optimizing botulinum toxin therapy for hyperhidrosis. Heckmann M et al. Br J Dermatol. 1998; 138: 553–4

Botulinum toxin in the treatment of palmar hyperhidrosis. Holmes S, Mann C. J Am Acad Dermatol. 1998; 39: 1040–1

Focal hyperhidrosis: effective treatment with intracutaneous botulinum toxin. Naumann M et al. Arch Dermatol. 1998; 134: 301–4

Botulinum toxin for focal hyperhidrosis: technical considerations and improvements in application. Naumann M et al. Br J Dermatol. 1998; 139: 1123–4

Hyperhidrosis treated by botulinum A exotoxin. Odderson IR. Dermatol Surg. 1998; 24: 1237–41

Botulinum toxin therapy for palmar hyperhidrosis. Shelley WB et al. J Am Acad Dermatol. 1998; 38: 227–9

[Treatment of hyperhidrosis by botulinum toxin]. Beaulieu P. Ann Dermatol Venereol. 1999; 126: 469–73

Side-controlled intradermal injection of botulinum toxin A in recalcitrant axillary hyperhidrosis. Heckmann M et al. J Am Acad Dermatol. 1999; 41: 987–90

12.4   Relative Hypersalivation

Sialorrhea in amyotrophic lateral sclerosis: a hypothesis of a new treatment–botulinum toxin A injections of the parotid glands. Bushara KO. Med Hypotheses 1997; 48: 337 – 9

Botulinum toxin is a useful treatment in excessive drooling in saliva. Bhatia KP et al. J Neurol Neurosurg Psychiatry 1999; 67: 697

12.5   Rhinorrhea

Rhinorrhea is decreased in dogs after nasal application of botulinum toxin. Shaari CM et al. Otolaryngol Head Neck Surg. 1995; 112: 566 – 71

Botulinum toxin and rhinorrhea [letter]. Bushara-KO. Otolaryngol Head Neck Surg. 1996; 114: 507

The effect of botulinum toxin type A injection for intrinsic rhinitis. Kim KS et al. J Laryngol Otol. 1998; 112: 248 – 51

13   Bladder Dysfunction
13.1   Detrusor Sphincter Dyssynergia

[Bladder dysfunctions in encephalomyelitis disseminata–drug and interventional therapeutic options]. Zwergel U et al. Fortschr Neurol Psychiatr. 1995; 63: 495 – 503

Botulinum-A toxin as a treatment of detrusor-sphincter dyssynergia: a prospective study in 24 spinal cord injury patients. Schurch B et al. J Urol. 1996; 155: 1023 – 9

Botulinum A toxin as a treatment of detrusor-sphincter dyssynergia in patients with spinal cord injury: MRI controlled transperineal injections. Schurch B et al. J Neurol Neurosurg Psychiatry 1997; 63: 474 – 6

Treatment of detrusor sphincter dyssynergia by transperineal injection of botulinum toxin. Gallien P et al. Arch Phys Med Rehabil. 1998; 79 : 715 – 7

Botulinum A toxin treatment for detrusor-sphincter dyssynergia in spinal cord disease. Petit H et al. Spinal Cord 1998; 36: 91 – 4

13.2   Bladder Sphincter Spasm

Botulinum toxin in the treatment of chronic urinary retention in women. Fowler CJ et al. Br J Urol. 1992; 70: 387 – 9

[Bladder dysfunctions in encephalomyelitis disseminata–drug and interventional therapeutic options]. Zwergel U et al. Fortschr Neurol Psychiatr. 1995; 63: 495 – 503

Botulinum toxin injections for voiding dysfunction following SCI. Wheeler JS Jr et al. J Spinal Cord Med. 1998; 21: 227 – 9

14 Various

14.1 Neurology

14.1.1 Tremor

Botulinum toxin treatment of tremors. Jankovic J, Schwartz K. Neurology 1991; 41: 1185–8

Botulinum toxin treatment of essential head tremor. Pahwa R. Neurology 1995; 45: 822–4

Yes/yes head tremor without appendicular tremor after bilateral cerebellar infarction. Finsterer J et al. J Neurol Sci. 1996; 139: 242–5

Botulinum toxin A in non-dystonic tremors. Henderson JM et al. Eur Neurol. 1996; 36: 29–35

A randomized, double-blind, placebo-controlled study to evaluate botulinum toxin type A in essential hand tremor. Jankovic J et al. Mov Disord. 1996; 11: 250–6

Quantitative assessment of botulinum toxin treatment in 43 patients with head tremor. Wissel J et al. Mov Disord. 1997; 12: 722–6

14.1.2 Tardive Dyskinesia

Botulinum toxin in treatment of tardive dyskinetic syndrome [letter]. Truong DD et al. J Clin Psychopharmacol. 1990; 10: 438–9

Botulinum toxin in a case of severe tardive dyskinesia mixed with dystonia [letter]. Stip E et al. Br J Psychiatry 1992; 161: 867–8

Complete remission of neuroleptic-induced Meige's syndrome by botulinum toxin treatment: a case report. Kurata K et al. Jpn J Psychiatry Neurol. 1993; 47: 115–9

Use of botulinum toxin injections for spasmodic torticollis of tardive dystonia. Kaufman DM. J Neuropsychiatry Clin Neurosci. 1994; 6: 50–3

Successful treatment of intractable tardive dyskinesia with botulinum toxin [letter]. Yasufuku-Takano J et al. J Neurol Neurosurg Psychiatry 1995; 58: 511–2

Improvement of both tardive dystonia and akathisia after botulinum toxin injection. Shulman LM et al. Neurology 1996; 46: 844–5

Treatment of facial and orolinguomandibular tardive dystonia by botulinum toxin A: evidence of a long-lasting effect. Kanovsky P et al. Mov Disord. 1999; 14: 886–8

14.1.3 Palatal Myoclonus

Ear click in palatal tremor: its origin and treatment with botulinum toxin. Deuschl G et al. Neurology 1991; 41: 1677–9

The use of clostridium botulinum toxin in palatal myoclonus. A preliminary report. Saeed SR, Brookes GB. J Laryngol Otol. 1993; 107: 208–10

Palatal myoclonus: treatment with Clostridium botulinum toxin injection. Varney SM et al. Otolaryngol Head Neck Surg. 1996; 114: 317–20

14.1.4 Gilles de la Tourette Syndrome

Botulinum toxin for refractory vocal tics. Salloway S et al. Mov Disord. 1996; 11: 746–8

Severe motor tics causing cervical myelopathy in Tourette's syndrome. Krauss JK, Jankovic J. Mov Disord. 1996; 11: 563–6

Botulinum toxin injection into vocal cord in the treatment of malignant coprolalia associated with Tourette's syndrome. Scott BL et al. Mov Disord. 1996; 11: 431–3

Vocal tics in Gilles de la Tourette syndrome treated with botulinum toxin injections. Trimble MR et al. Mov Disord. 1998; 13: 617–9

Tics in Tourette syndrome: new treatment options. Awaad Y. J Child Neurol. 1999; 14: 316–9

14.1.5 Myoclonus

Effectiveness of botulinum toxin type A against painful limb myoclonus of spinal cord origin. Polo KB, Jabbari B. Mov Disord. 1994; 9: 233–5

Treatment of childhood myoclonus with botulinum toxin type A. Awaad Y et al. Child Neurol. 1999; 14: 781–6

Stimulus-sensitive spinal segmental myoclonus improved with injections of botulinum toxin type A. Lagueny A et al. Mov Disord. 1999; 14: 182–5

14.1.6 Pain

Botulinum toxin in the treatment of myofascial pain syndrome. Cheshire WP et al. Pain. 1994; 59: 65–9

Use of botulinum toxin to alleviate facial pain [letter]. Girdler NM. Br J Hosp Med. 1994; 52: 363

Botulinum toxin in painful syndromes. Monsivais JJ, Monsivais DB. Hand Clin. 1996; 12: 787–9

Botulinum toxin is unsatisfactory therapy for fibromyalgia. Paulson GW, Gill W. Mov Disord. 1996; 11: 459

Botulinum toxin injection for cervicogenic headache. Hobson DE, Gladish DF. Headache 1997; 37: 253–5

14.1.7 Stiff Person Syndrome

Significant improvement of stiff-person syndrome after paraspinal injection of botulinum toxin A. Davis D, Jabbari B. Mov Disord. 1993; 8: 371–3

Botulinum toxin A improves muscle spasms and rigidity in stiff-person syndrome. Liguori R et al. Mov Disord. 1997; 12: 1060–3

14.1.8 Myokymia

Intractable orbicularis myokymia: treatment alternatives. Jordan DR et al. Ophthalmic-Surg. 1989; 20: 280–3

14.1.9 Tetanus

Botulinum toxin A for trismus in cephalic tetanus. Andrade LA, Brucki SM. Arq Neuropsiquiatr. 1994; 52: 410–3

14.1.10 Rigidity

Botulinum toxin-A improves the rigidity of progressive supranuclear palsy. Polo KB, Jabbari B. Ann Neurol. 1994; 35: 237 – 9

14.1.11 Benign Muscle Cramps

Botulinum toxin treatment of muscle cramps: a clinical and neurophysiological study. Bertolasi L et al. Ann Neurol. 1997; 41: 181 – 6

14.1.12 Dopa-Associated Dyskinesias

"Off" painful dystonia in Parkinson's disease treated with botulinum toxin. Pacchetti C et al. Mov Disord. 1995; 10: 333 – 6

14.1.13 Paradoxic Jaw Muscle Activity

Botulinum toxin in the management of paradoxical activity of jaw muscles [letter]. Naumann M et al. J Neurol Neurosurg Psychiatry 1995; 59: 192 – 3

14.1.14 Hereditary Chin Trembling

Treatment of hereditary trembling chin with botulinum toxin. Bakar M et al. Mov Disord. 1998; 13: 845 – 6

14.1.15 Hemimasticatory Spasm

Hemimasticatory spasm in hemifacial atrophy: diagnostic and therapeutic aspects in two patients. Ebersbach G et al. Mov Disord. 1995; 10: 504 – 7

14.1.16 Maseteric Hypertrophy

The medical management of masseteric hypertrophy with botulinum toxin type A. Moore AP, Wood GD. Br J Oral Maxillofac Surg. 1994; 32: 26 – 8
Botulinum toxin treatment of bilateral masseteric hypertrophy. Smyth AG. Br J Oral Maxillofac Surg. 1994; 32: 29 – 33

14.1.17 Hypertrophic Branchial Myopathy

Hypertrophic branchial myopathy treated with botulinum toxin type A. Doyle M, Jabbari B. Neurology 1994; 44: 1765 – 6

14.1.18 Tibialis Anterior Hypertrophy

Persistent unilateral tibialis anterior muscle hypertrophy with complex repetitive discharges and myalgia: report of two unique cases and response to botulinum toxin [see comments]. Nix WA et al. Neurology 1992; 42: 602 – 6

14.1.19 Nystagmus

Management of symptomatic latent nystagmus. Liu C et al. Eye 1993; 7: 550 – 3
The use of botulinum toxin for treatment of acquired nystagmus and oscillopsia. Ruben ST et al. Ophthalmology 1994; 101: 783 – 7
The treatment of congenital nystagmus with Botox. Carruthers J. J Pediatr Ophthalmol Strabismus. 1995; 32: 306 – 8

Unsatisfactory treatment of acquired nystagmus with retrobulbar injection of botulinum toxin. Tomsak RL et al. Am J Ophthalmol. 1995; 119: 489 – 96

Cosmetic therapy with botulinum toxin, Anecdotal memoirs. Klein AW. Dermatol Surg. 1996; 22: 757 – 9

Periodic alternating nystagmus treated with retrobulbar botulinum toxin and large horizontal muscle recession. Thomas R et al. Indian J Ophthalmol. 1996; 44: 170 – 2

14.1.20 Oscillopsia

Retrobulbar botulinum toxin for treatment of oscillopsia. Ruben S et al. Aust NZ J Ophthalmol. 1994; 22: 65 – 7

The use of botulinum toxin for treatment of acquired nystagmus and oscillopsia. Ruben ST et al. Ophthalmology 1994; 101: 783 – 7

14.1.21 Supranuclear Gaze Palsy

Botulinum toxin treatment of supranuclear ocular motility disorders. Newman NJ, Lambert SR. Neurology 1992; 42: 1391 – 3

Botulinum toxin treatment of Hertwig-Magendie sign. Rebolleda G, Munoz Negrete FJ. Eur J Ophthalmol. 1996; 6: 217 – 9

14.1.22 Epilepsia Partialis Continua

Botulinum toxin treatment is not effective for epilepsy partialis continua [letter]. Tarsy D, Schachter SC. Mov Disord. 1995; 10: 357 – 8

14.1.23 Operation Planning

Selective peripheral denervation for spasmodic torticollis: is the outcome predictable? Braun V et al. J Neurol. 1995; 242: 504 – 7

14.2 Otorhinolaryngology

14.2.1 Abductor Vocal Cord Paralysis

Use of botulinum toxin to lateralize true vocal cords: a biochemical method to relieve bilateral abductor vocal cord paralysis. Cohen SR, Thompson JW. Ann Otol Rhinol Laryngol. 1987; 96: 534 – 41

Botulinum toxin for relief of bilateral abductor paralysis of the larynx: histologic study in an animal model. Cohen SR et al. Ann Otol Rhinol Laryngol. 1989; 98: 213 – 6

14.2.2 Recalcitant Mutational Dysphonia

Botulinum toxin in the treatment of recalcitrant mutational dysphonia. Woodson GE, Murry T. J Voice 1994; 8: 347 – 51

14.2.3 Upper Oesophageal Sphincter Dysfunction

Treatment of dysfunction of the cricopharyngeal muscle with botulinum A toxin: introduction of a new, noninvasive method. Schneider I et al. Ann Otol Rhinol Laryngol. 1994; 103: 31 – 5

14.2.4 Vocal Fold Granuloma

Treatment of vocal fold granuloma using botulinum toxin type A. Nasri S et al. Laryngoscope 1995; 105: 585 – 8

14.2.5 Stuttering

Laryngeal botulinum toxin injections for disabling stuttering in adults. Brin MF et al. Neurology 1994; 44: 2262 – 6

Activity of intrinsic laryngeal muscles in fluent and disfluent speech. Smith A et al. J Speech Hear Res. 1996; 39: 329 – 48

14.2.6 Middle Ear Myoclonus

Management of middle ear myoclonus. Badia L et al. J Laryngol Otol. 1994; 108: 380 – 2

14.2.7 Protective Larynx Closure

Repeatedly successful closure of the larynx for the treatment of chronic aspiration with the use of botulinum toxin A. Pototschnig CA et al. Ann Otol Rhinol Laryngol. 1996; 105: 521 – 4

14.2.8 Postlaryngectomy Speech Failure

Voice failure after tracheoesophageal puncture: management with botulinum toxin. Blitzer A et al. Otolaryngol Head Neck Surg. 1995; 113: 668 – 70

Botulinum toxin injection for postlaryngectomy tracheoesophageal speech failure. Terrell JE et al. Otolaryngol Head Neck Surg. 1995; 113: 788 – 91

Using botulinum toxin A to improve speech and swallowing function following total laryngectomy. Crary MA, Glowasky AL. Arch Otolaryngol Head Neck Surg. 1996; 122: 760

14.3 Ophthalmology

14.3.1 Protective Ptosis

Botulinum toxin A induced protective ptosis. Adams GG et al. Eye 1987; 1: 603 – 8

Botulinum toxin A-induced protective ptosis in corneal disease. Kirkness CM et al. Ophthalmology 1988; 95: 473 – 80

Therapeutic ptosis with botulinum toxin in epikeratoplasty. Freegard T et al. Br J Ophthalmol. 1993; 77: 820 – 2

Management of superior limbic keratoconjunctivitis with botulinum toxin [letter]. Mackie IA. Eye 1995; 9: 143 – 4

Protective ptosis after parotid surgery induced with botulinum toxin. Smyth AG. Br J Oral Maxillofac Surg. 1995; 33: 107 – 9

[Protective ptosis by botulinum A toxin injection in corneal affectations]. Gusek-Schneider GC, Erbguth F. Klin Monatsbl Augenheilkd. 1998; 213: 15 – 22

14.3.2 Entropion

Botulinum toxin for benign essential blepharospasm, hemifacial spasm and age-related lower eyelid entropion. Carruthers J, Stubbs HA. Can J Neurol Sci. 1987; 14: 42 – 5

Botulinum A-toxin treatment of spasmodic entropion of the lower eyelid. Neetens A et al. Bull Soc Belge Ophtalmol. 1987; 224: 105 – 9

Treatment of senile entropion with botulinum toxin. Clarke JR, Spalton DJ. Br J Ophthalmol. 1988; 72: 361 – 2

Botulinum toxin type A in upper lid retraction of Graves' ophthalmopathy. Ebner R. J Clin Neuroophthalmol. 199; 13: 258 – 61

14.4 Gastroenterology

14.4.1 Sphincter Odii Dysfunction

[Diagnostic and therapeutic possibilities in suspected Oddi's sphincter dysfunction]. Wehrmann T et al. Z Gastroenterol. 1994; 32: 694 – 701

Effects of botulinum toxin A on the sphincter of Oddi: an in vivo and in vitro study. Sand J et al. Gut 1998; 42: 507 – 10

Endoscopic injection of botulinum toxin for biliary sphincter of Oddi dysfunction. Wehrmann T et al. Endoscopy 1998; 30: 702 – 7

Endoscopic botulinum toxin injection into the minor papilla for treatment of idiopathic recurrent pancreatitis in patients with pancreas divisum. Wehrmann T et al. Endoscopy 1999; 50: 545 – 8

14.4.2 Coeliac Plexus Blockade

Percutaneous celiac plexus block with botulinum toxin A did not help the pain of chronic pancreatitis. Sherman S et al. J Clin-Gastroenterol. 1995; 20: 343 – 4

14.4.3 Pseudoachalasia

Botulinum toxin for suspected pseudoachalasia. Vallera RA, Brazer SR. Am J Gastroenterol. 1995; 90: 1319 – 21

14.4.4 Nonachalasia Oesophageal Motor Disorders

Treatment of symptomatic nonachalasia esophageal motor disorders with botulinum toxin injection at the lower esophageal sphincter. Miller LS et al. Dig Dis Sci. 1996; 41: 2025 – 31

14.5 Gynaecology

14.5.1 Vaginismus

Treatment of vaginismus with botulinum toxin injections [letter]. Brin MF, Vapnek JM. Lancet 1997; 349: 252 – 3

14.6 Urology

14.6.1 Prostate Hyperplasia

Botox-induced prostatic involution. Doggweiler R et al. Prostate 1998; 37: 44 – 50

Relief by botulinum toxin of voiding dysfunction due to prostatitis. Maria G et al. Lancet 1998; 352: 625

14.7 Surgery

14.7.1 Anismus

Initial North American experience with botulinum toxin type A for treatment of anismus. Joo JS et al. Dis Colon Rectum 1996; 39: 1107 – 11

Severe constipation in Parkinson's disease relieved by botulinum toxin. Albanese A et al. Mov Disord. 1997; 12: 764 – 6

14.8 Orthopaedic Surgery

14.8.1 Postoperative Immobilisation

Botulinum toxin A in orthopaedic surgery [letter]. Gasser T et al. Lancet 1991; 338: 761

Botulinum toxin enhancement of postoperative immobilization in patients with cervical dystonia. Technical note. Traynelis VC et al. J Neurosurg. 1992; 77: 808 – 9

Selective peripheral denervation for the treatment of spasmodic torticollis. Braun V, Richter HP. Neurosurgery 1994; 35: 58 – 62; discussion 62 – 3

Preoperative treatment with botulinum toxin to facilitate cervical fusion in dystonic cerebral palsy. Report of two cases. Racette BA et al. J Neurosurg. 1998; 88: 328 – 30

Addresses

This list contains the addresses of patient support groups, professional organisations, professional journals, as well as the manufacturers and distributors of botulinum toxin arranged according to country.

Australia

Australian Spasmodic
Torticollis Association
c/o Annette Walker
PO Box 133
Westmead
New South Wales, 2145
Australia
phone: +61-296-859-020
fax: +61-296-859-599
email: a.walker@uws.edu.au

Belgium

Belgische Zelphulpgroep Voor
Dystonie Patiënten
c/o Christine Wauters
Blokmakerstraat 6
9120 Haasdonk
Belgium
phone: +32-3-7755125
fax: +32-3-7755125

Brazil

Associação Brasileira
dos Portadores de Distonias
c/o Elenita Ferreira de Macedo
Al. Santos, 1780 13 andar
São Paolo, SP Cep: 01448-200
Brazil
phone: +55-112871264
fax: +55-112871264

Chile

Fundacion Distonia
c/o Benedicte De Pauw
Av. Irarrazaral 5185, Of. 311
Nunoa, Santiago
Chile
phone: +56-22 26 88 74
fax: +56-22 26 73 46

Croatia

Hrvatska Grupa Za Istrazivanje
Distonije
c/o Prof. Maja Relja
University of Zagreb
Kispaticeva 12
Zagreb, 10000
Croatia
phone: +385-01-233-5595
fax: +385-01-233-5595

Denmark

Dansk Dystoniforening
c/o Ulla Balser Poulsen
Solhojpark 16
3520 Farum
Denmark
phone: +45-4295-5165
fax: +45-4295-5165
email: ullafarum@teliamail.dk
website: http://www.dystoni.dk

France

Association de Malades
atteints de Dystonie (AMADYS)
c/o Marcel Besse
20 rue de la Cote du Theil
03310 Lavault Sainte Anne
France
phone: + 33-470-291-771
fax: + 33-470-291-771
email: amadys@wanadoo.fr
website: http://perso.wanadoo.fr
            /amadys

Ligue Française contre la Dystonie
27 rue du Bout des Creuses
91210 Draveil
France
phone: + 33-169 83 23 39
fax: + 33-169 83 23 39
email: lfcd@wanadoo.fr
website: http://perso.wanadoo.fr
            /lfcd

Finland

Finnish Dystonia Association
c/o Liisi Niemi
Ostjakinkatu 5 as 29
20750 Turku
Finland
email: liisi.niemi@pp.inet.fi
website: personal.inet.fi/koti/
            liisi.niemi/
            Finndystonia.html

Germany

Bundesverband Torticollis e.V.
c/o Helga Weber
Eckernkamp 39
59077 Hamm
Germany
phone: + 49-2389-53 69 88
fax: + 49-2389-53 62 89
email: BVTorti@aol.com

Deutsche Dystonie
Gesellschaft e.V.
c/o Didi Jackson
Bockhorst 45 A
22589 Hamburg
Germany
phone: + 49-40-870 21 33
fax: + 49-40-87 56 02
email: Deutsche-Dystonie
            @t-online.de
website: http://www.
            dystonie.de

Elan Pharma GmbH
c/o Dr. Bernd Sierakowski
Rosenkavallierplatz 8
81925 München
phone: + 49-89-99 99 70 31
fax: + 49-89-99 99 70 41
email: bsierakowski@elan-
            pharma.de

Merz & Co.
Eckenheimer Landstr. 100 – 104
60318 Frankfurt/Main
Germany
phone: + 49-69-15 03-1
fax: + 49-69-59 97 78
email: merzpr@merz.de
website: http://www.merz.de

Great Britain

Elan Pharmaceuticals Europe
c/o Timothy H. Corn
Elan House
Avenue One
Letchworth
Herts SG6 2HU
United Kingdom
phone: + 44-1462-707-200
fax: + 44-1462-707-253
email: TimCorn@ElanEurope.
           com

European Dystonia
Federation (EDF)
c/o The Dystonia Society
46 – 47 Britton Street
London ECIM 5NA
United Kingdom
phone: + 44-171-490-5671
fax: + 44-171-490-5672

Headway
National Head Injury Association
7 King Edwards Court
King Edward Street
Nottingham NG1 1EW
United Kingdom
phone: + 44-1159-224-0800

Ipsen Ltd.
1 Bath Road
Maidenhead
Berkshire SL6 4UH
United Kingdom
phone: + 44-1628-771417
fax: + 44-1628-770211
email: medinfo@ipsen.ltd.uk
website: http://www.ipsen.
           ltd.uk

Multiple Sclerosis Society
of Great Britain and
Northern Ireland
25 Effie Road
London SW6 1EE
United Kingdom
phone: + 44-171-736-627

SCOPE
c/o Richard Parnell
6 Market Road
London N7 9PW
United Kingdom
phone: + 44-171-619-7258
fax: + 44-171-619-7380
email: richard.parnell@scope.
           org.uk
website: http://www.scope.
           org.uk

Spinal Injuries Association
Newpoint House
St James's Lane
London N10 3 DF
United Kingdom
phone: + 44-181-444-2121

The Dystonia Society (TDS)
46 – 47 Britton Street
London ECIM 5NA
United Kingdom
phone: + 44-171-490-5671
fax: + 44-171-490-5672

The Stroke Association
CHSA House
123 – 127 Whitecross Street
London EC1 Y 8JJ
United Kingdom
phone: + 44-171-490-7999

Ireland

The Dystonia Society in Ireland
c/o Maria Hickey
33 Larkfield Grove-Harold Cross
Dublin 6 W
Republic of Ireland
phone: + 353-196-4387

Italy

Assoc. Italiana per la Ricerca
Sulla Distonia
c/o Anna Florenzani
Via Arturo Colautti 28
00152 Rome
Italy
phone: + 39-06-589-8727
fax: + 39-06-580-3940
email: segreteria.ard@iol.it
website: http://www.web
            zone.it/distonia

Japan

Dystonia Support Group of Japan
c/o Masako Kaji
Ohtsu Central Post Office Box 11
Ohtsu City
520 Shiga
Japan
phone: + 81-775-330-297
fax: + 81-775-379-753

New Zealand

New Zealand Spasmodic
Dysphonia Patients' Network
15 Pluto Place
North Shore City
Auckland 1310
New Zealand

phone: + 64-9-482-1567
fax: + 64-9-482-1284
email: dsbarton@ihug.co.nz

Norway

Norsk Dystoniforening
c/o Tore Wirgenes
PO Box 1545 Glombo
1677 Krakeroy
Norge
phone: + 47-35 02 05 38
fax: + 47-35 01 39 60
website: http://www.home.sol.
            no/torwi

Slovenia

Dystonia Association of Slovenia
c/o Dr. Zvezdan Pirtosek
Instit. of Clinical Neurophysiology
University Medical Centre
1525 Ljubljana
Slovenia
phone: + 38-661-316-152
fax: + 38-661-302-771

South Africa

South African Dystonia
Association
c/o Maureen Langford
PO Box 3160
2123s Pinegowrie
South Africa
phone: + 27-11-7878792
fax: + 27-11-7878792
email: parkins@global.co.za

Spain

Asoc. de Lucha contra
la Distonia en España
c/o Felisa Justo Alonso
c/ Galileo, 69-1
28015 Madrid
Spain
phone: + 34-91-7598866
fax: + 34-91-7598866
email: alde@mx3.redestb.es
website: http://www.arrakis.es/
~amolina/alde.htm

Sweden

Svensk Dystoni Forening
c/o Anders Silfors
Stjarngossevagen 108
12535 Alvsjo
Sweden
phone: + 46-8999956
fax: + 46-8999956
website: http://www.patient
information.com/
www.pion.et

Switzerland

Schweizerische Dystonie
Gesellschaft (SDG)
Tramstr. 39
4132 Muttenz
Switzerland
phone: + 41-6146-16993
fax: + 41-6146-16993

The Netherlands

Nederlandse Verening
van Dystoniepatienten
c/o Louis Beduwe
Postbus 9345
4801 LH Breda
The Netherlands
phone: + 31-76-522-7548
fax: + 31-76-521-6495

United States of America

Allergan Inc.
2525 Dupont Drive
PO Box 15934
Irvine
CA 92713-9534
USA
phone: + 1-714-253-5413
fax: + 1-714-752-4359
email: corpinfo@allergan.com
website: http://www.allergan.
com

American Academy of Neurology
1080 Montreal Avenue
St. Paul
MN 55116
USA
phone: + 1-651-695-1940
email: web@aan.com
website: http://www.aan.com

American Neurological
Association
5841 Cedar Lake Road
Suite #204
Minneapolis
MN 55416
USA

phone: + 1-612-545-62 84
fax: + 1-612-545-60 73
email: ewilkerson@compu-
serve.com
website: http://www.aneuroa.
org

Benign Essential Blepharospasm
Research Foundation, Inc.
c/o Mary Lou Thompson
P. O. Box 12468
Beaumont
TX 77726-2468
USA
phone: + 1-409-832-0788
fax: + 1-409-832-0890
email: bebrf@ih2000.net
website: http://www.
blepharospasm.org

Dystonia Medical Research
Foundation
One East Wacker Drive
Suite 2430
Chicago
IL 60601-1905
USA
phone: + 1-312-755-0198
fax: + 1-312-803-0138
email: dystonia@dystonia-
foundation.org
website: http://www.dystonia-
foundation.org

Elan Pharmaceuticals
c/o Dr. David Mason
800 Gateway Boulevard
South San Francisco
CA 94080
USA
phone: + 1-650-794-5743
fax: + 1-650-553-7150
email: dmason@elanpharma.
com

International Tremor Foundation
c/o Catherine Rice
7046 West 105th Street
Overland Park
KS 66212-1803
USA
phone: + 1-888-387-3667
fax: + 1-913-341-1296
email: inttremorfndn@world
net.att.net
website: http://www.essential
tremor.org

Movement Disorders
Lippincott Williams & Wilkins
P. O. Box 1600
Hagerstown
MD 21740-1600
USA
phone: + 1-301-714-23 34
fax: + 1-301-824-23 65
website: http://www.lww.com

National Spasmodic Dysphonia
Association (NSDA)
One East Wacker Drive
Suite 2430
Chicago
IL 60601-1905
USA
phone: +1-312-755-0198
fax: +1-312-803-0138
email: dystonia@dystonia-
         foundation.org
website: http://www.dystonia-
         foundation.org

National Spasmodic Torticollis
Association (NSTA)
9920 Talbert Avenue, Suite 233
Fountain Valley
CA 92708
USA
phone: +1-714-378-7838
fax: +1-714-378-7830
website: http://www.torticollis.
         org

Our Voice
National SD Newsletter
Suite 13E
365 W 25th Street
New York
NY 10001-5816
USA
phone: +1-212-929-4299
fax: +1-212-929-4099

Tardive Dyskinesia/Tardive
Dystonia National Association
PO Box 45732
Seattle
WA 98145-0732
USA
phone: +1-206-522-3166

The Bachmann-Strauss Dystonia
& Parkinson Foundation, Inc.
c/o Bonnie Strauss
1 Gustave L. Levy Place
Box 1490
New York
NY 10029
USA
phone: +1-212-241-5614
fax: +1-212-987-0662
email: Bachmann.Strauss
         @mssm.edu
website: http://www.dystonia-
         parkinsons.org

The Movement Disorders Society
Secretariat
611 Wells Street
Milwaukee
WI 53202
USA
phone: +1-414-276-2145
fax: +1-414-276-2146
email: KStanton@movement
         disorders.org
website: http://www.movement
         disorders.org

We Move
204 West 84th Street
New York
NY 10024
USA
phone: +1-212-875-8312
fax: +1-212-875-8389
email: wemove@wemove.org
website: http://www.wemove.
         org

Index